Collapsed Lung
Causes and
Symptoms

The ideas, information and suggestions in this book are purely the ideas of the author and are not substitutes for consulting your physician. We will not accept responsibility for any action or claim resulting from the use of information contained in this book.

First published in 2017 by Reklaw Education Limited

Collapsed Lung

Causes and Symptoms

Joseph Appleton

REKLAW EDUCATION (UK)

Foreword

Every year, millions of people suffer from Collapsed Lung (or 'Pneumothorax') in the Unites States, the United Kingdom and elsewhere.

There are very few resources about Collapsed Lung that offer detailed information for public awareness. This book offers everything that you should know about Collapsed Lung.

We highlight the most common causes and symptoms of the disease with patient profiles to give readers a clear understanding about life with Collapsed Lung. The earlier sections of the book discuss the causes, symptoms and possible treatments for the disease. In addition, a separate section has been dedicated towards useful resources for patients and family members to help them through the after-surgery healing process.

Researchers have identified various factors that might cause primary or secondary Pneumothorax. This book discusses various past and recent developments regarding Pneumothorax to help readers understand the disease better. The latter sections of the book offer a comprehensive guide that aims to help patients deal with the disease. Readers can read patient profiles and learn about the treatment and prevention of the disease before it causes any damage.

Acknowledgements

These acknowledgements on paper are in no way reflective or representative of the actual depth of my feelings of gratitude to the people who have made the publication of this book possible. Ever since I was a child I have dreamt of one thing, to be able to help others in one way or another. This drive has pushed me to not only write this book but to also acknowledge the driving forces behind this ambition to help people. It is a testament to a person's parents and their upbringing when they grow into someone who helps other human beings. This is why I am most thankful to my parents whose efforts in my childhood, patience in my adolescence, understanding in my youth and guidance in my adulthood has given me the courage and the perseverance to continue on with my dreams.

A big thank you to all who have been a contributing factor in this book; whether in a large capacity or small, your efforts have made this possible just as much as mine.

Thank you!

Joseph Appleton

Contents

What Is Collapsed Lung?

Collapsed Lung is a breathing condition, medically known as Pneumothorax. This complicated term is derived from two words; Pneumo, meaning air and Thorax, meaning chest cavity. Many a time, this condition is a result of injuries to the upper abdomen; however, several cases of Collapsed Lung have been reported world over that do not involve any severe injuries. Hence, many doctors describe its 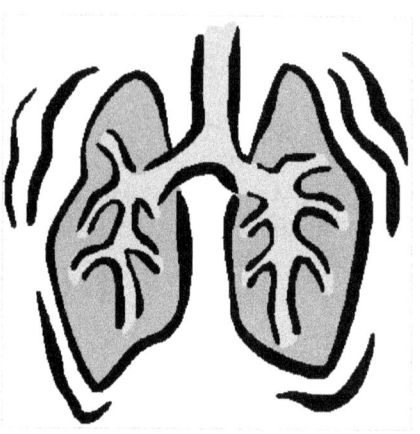 occurrence as 'out of the blue' in healthy young people; in which case it is called Spontaneous Pneumothorax.

A more detailed analysis of Collapsed Lung suggests that while the individual may be healthy and young, even a small tear on the outer surface of the lungs can result in this condition. This tear may be a result of exertion or intense activity as well. Despite this diagnosis, the causes of a lung collapse are often vague and puzzling if no apparent exertion or injury is reported.

Pneumothorax is characterized by the leakage of air from the lungs. To completely understand this condition, a review detailing the functions of the lungs is in order. Oxygen usually enters the lungs *via* the trachea. Also known as the windpipe, the trachea branches out into two main pipes, each leading into one lung. These pipes are called Bronchi.

Each Bronchus branches out into a bronchial tree, called a Bronchial system that is made up of delicate tube like structures. A large number of tubes in the lungs ensure that adequate oxygen is delivered here. Once air reaches the lungs, it is delivered to all other body parts and other organs by being absorbed into the blood stream.

Collapsed lungs are a serious ailment that affect the ability of these vital organs to function properly. The entire body suffers as a result since every part relies on the lungs for the essential supply of air. When air leaks from within the lungs, it fills the surrounding space between the lungs and the chest wall called the Pleural Space, causing the lungs to collapse as a result. This happens because the added pressure prevents them from expanding to their full potential. In many severe cases, the collapsing effect is so intense that the lungs are pushed down; making it very hard for the patient to breath normally.

The severity of Pneumothorax varies from case to case. In most scenarios, the lungs collapse in sections; affecting one part while the remaining stays intact to supply oxygen to the body. Depending on how severe the collapse is, medical treatment varies. In many minor cases, the trapped air soon leaves the system, helping the lungs regain their shape and functionality. In others, a complicated surgery is the only way to relieve pain and restore lung function.

A collapsed lung also results in many other serious ailments if it is left untreated for too long. Since the trapped air puts tremendous pressure on the lungs and the heart, it can result in cardiac stress and in severe cases, cardiac arrest as well. Therefore, doctors suggest that every case of Pneumothorax should be diagnosed and checked thoroughly even if it is a minor one.

Types of Collapsed Lungs

Knowing the types of Collapsed Lung is an important step towards recognizing its symptoms and preparing for treatment. A Pneumothorax that is minor in nature often goes undetected because a lot of people confuse its symptoms with every day uneasiness or health issues that come and go with time. This is why, understanding the fine details of this ailment is not only necessary, it is highly crucial to take prompt notice.

As mentioned previously, a collapsed lung can occur in injured patients as well as healthy individuals. While the rate of occurrence with an injury is higher, the timing, severity and lasting effect are some of the main differentiating factors by which the various types of Pneumothorax are classified.

Predominantly, there are two types of Pneumothorax. Both are treated differently and their symptoms and effects vary as well.

1. **Traumatic Pneumothorax (TP)**

    Traumatic Pneumothorax is a more severe kind of lung collapse that occurs after a person suffers from an injury. Such an injury is usually directed towards the chest and upper abdomen. Meeting with an accident or taking a sharp fall are some instances in which intense damage to the lungs can result in the leakage of air from the sac.

    Moreover, many a time, Pneumothorax is also a result of severe shock and pressured breathing during which the lungs can develop a tear in their outer lining. This usually happens when the lungs cannot keep pace with the body's need for increased oxygen supply.

    Other examples of Traumatic Lung Damage are:

    - A deep stab to the chest, resulting in an open wound.

    - Sudden impact with air bags in the case of an accident.

    - Hitting the chest during contact sports like Rugby.

- Intense medical procedures that affect the functionality of the lungs. These include prolonged use of ventilators, insertion of chest tubes and lung biopsies.

Since TP includes wounds, pain and bodily damage, treating it promptly is necessary to contain bleeding and take pressure off the lungs.

2. Non-Traumatic Pneumothorax (NTP)

Non-Traumatic Pneumothorax has been mentioned lightly in the previous discussion. Such a case of lung collapse is the opposite of TP, i.e. it occurs spontaneously and does not follow only after an injury. Within the NTP category, there are three types of lung collapses.

- Primary Spontaneous Pneumothorax (PSP) - As the name suggests, PSP occurs in patients for whom this is their first instance of a lung condition. These patients have never been diagnosed with any type of lung disease.

- Secondary Spontaneous Pneumothorax (SSP) – For a patient to be diagnosed with SSP, they should already have some kind of lung disease. SSP occurs in conjunction with this disease, which makes the condition more critical. Some lung related disorders that make a patient prone to SSP are lung cancer, cystic fibrosis, chronic infection, asthma and pulmonary obstructive disease.

- Spontaneous hemopneumothorax (SHP) – Compared to PSP and SSP, SHP is a relatively rare condition in which air and blood both fill the pleural cavity, making it impossible for the individual to breathe normally. What makes SHP fatal is that it can occur in the absence of any known lung disease as well.

How Common Is It? Factors Affecting Collapsed Lungs

Just like every disease is dependent on a host of factors, the occurrence and severity of a collapsed lung is also determined by many things. However, unlike other many common ailments, Pneumothorax can often result in the absence of prior symptoms or lung disease, thereby not only making it a dangerous condition, but also one that has to be watched out for consciously.

Who is more prone to lung collapse, at what age and with what type of health conditions? These are some questions that every layman should be well versed with because the minute lung collapse occurs, the signs are such that they do not attract immediate attention. That said, the condition under question can affect the daily working of an individual's body, crippling him from performing everyday tasks.

Therefore, it certainly helps to know the risk factors associated with Collapsed Lung, at least to an extent that if the condition occurs spontaneously, you recognize its occurrence and rush to an Emergency Room.

The different types of Pneumothorax have different risk factors because of how they occur. Since each type has a unique condition attached to it, it is safe to say that each type occurs in people who are most prone to its specific risk factors. Apart from the risk factors, many people question medical professionals regarding the commonality of this ailment.

While Traumatic Pneumothorax is almost always related to chest injury, PSP occurs without any rhyme or reason in individuals who have no lung disease either. Therefore, Collapsed Lung is quite common and is one of those ailments that take patients by surprise.

Risk Factors of Collapsed Lung

For Traumatic Pneumothorax, the risk factors include:

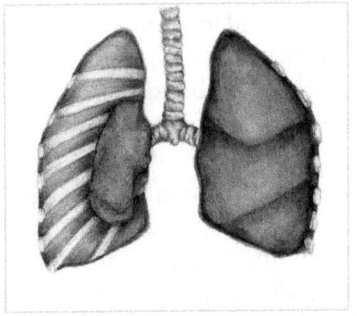

- A history of violence or street fighting that has resulted in multiple injuries time and again. Such behavior makes a person highly prone to developing a tear in the lung sack, which leads to collection of air in the chest cavity. It should be remembered that lung collapse, in conjunction with other head and abdomen injuries can turn into a highly dangerous and risky condition that can take a long while to fix.

- Involvement in contact sports on a regular basis. Rugby and wrestling are examples of such sporting activities that can result in vigorous blows to the chest and lung area. Performers who do stunts that put too much pressure on the chest cavity are also prone to developing Pneumothorax.

For Primary Spontaneous Pneumothorax, the risk factors are very diverse. Since this kind of condition results in people who have had no medical history of lung disease experiencing the onset of lung collapse; its sudden and unprecedented. It usually occurs while the person is resting or sleeping. Men aged 20 to 40 are the most prone to PSP and are diagnosed with varying degrees of the condition depending on their overall health.

Extensive studies have shown that PSP affects men six times more than women; especially those who are thin, tall and within the age bracket specified. Another risk factor that is the most common among PSP patients is smoking. Smokers are at a high risk of developing this condition because chain smoking results in the bursting of small bleb-like structures that are present on the side of each lung.

When these structures burst due to smoking, air is leaked into the chest cavity causing a Pneumothorax instantly. This should be taken as a warning sign by the smoker that their body is reacting to their bad habit

11

in the most negative manner. Hence, there can be no better time to quit smoking than in the aftermath of a sudden PSP attack. PSP also occurs in these males who are exposed to harsh environmental conditions or occupational factors like Silicosis.

For Secondary Spontaneous Pneumothorax, the risk factors are related to disease and chronic health issues. Since SSP is spurred on in the presence of lung disease or any other kind of serious ailments, its onset is magnified because of a compounded effect. If the disease has been diagnosed for quite some time, persistent coughing and heavy breathing can weaken the lung walls.

When this happens, the chances of developing a tear and leaking air into the chest cavity increase tremendously. As a result, SSP is usually seen in patients who are over 40 years of age and have been through some rough times concerning their health. Particular risk factors (diseases) that can cause SSP are:

• Pneumonia

• Cystic fibrosis

• Sarcoidosis

• Tuberculosis

• Idiopathic pulmonary fibrosis

• Lung cancer

In a nutshell, a patient's age, sex, medical history and general everyday habits are prominent risk factors that need to be considered when a diagnosis is made for Pneumothorax.

Facts and Statistics

Medical research has led to the collection of many facts and figures regarding Collapsed Lung. According to many medical professionals, Pneumothorax is not a very common disease, especially in its primary form. While traumatic and secondary nature lung collapses are seen in people, the former is a rare condition that affects 2 in 10,000 people in the United Kingdom on an annual basis.

On the whole, there is a 25% chance of recurrence in patients who have gone through one episode of Pneumothorax, and every 3 in 10 patients are likely to experience another instance of this condition within the first 6 months of being treated. This risk lasts for another three years, after which the lungs are completely repaired.

Following these statistics, patients who have gone through any type of Pneumothorax are advised to slow down their pace of life. Extensive travel and change of environmental conditions are discouraged so that the lungs are not put under added stress.

The occurrence of Primary Spontaneous Pneumothorax has been a topic of debate and extensive research lately. Observations have concluded that most of these cases are reported in young men who are experiencing rapid growth spurts. It is because of a sudden increase of their height and lean figure that the lung tear becomes prominent, leading to a collapse.

Clinics in the United States have been receiving 3 to 5 cases of lung collapse on a weekly basis, with all patients being young males. Apart from just a tall frame, the second most common reason is chain smoking. Almost 91% of those who experienced sharp pains in their chest, the biggest sign of a Pneumothorax, are smokers and have been so for some years. Men who smoke at least 20 cigarettes a day are to a 100-fold increase in the rate of occurrence of Pneumothorax.

In 2012, it was estimated that 226,000 people would be diagnosed with Lung Cancer, making the chances of a secondary lung collapse even higher. Among these people, 80% of those who do not survive, have tobacco to blame for their lung conditions. Therefore, smoking is the single most dangerous risk factor for lung cancer and eventual lung collapse in the most severe manner.

As mentioned previously, Collapsed Lung is a condition more common in men than women. In terms of the Annual Age Adjusted Incidence Rate, in every 100,000 people, the ratio for men and women patients is 7.4 : 1.2, and within the same population, the instance of Pneumothorax is up to 200 cases, if the individual is over 1.93 meters tall.

On a more positive note, death from Primary Spontaneous Pneumothorax alone is uncommon, provided that the overall health of the patient is intact. According to many combined statistics, the annual mortality rate in men is 1.26 deaths per million and in women, 0.62 deaths per million.

Patient Profile

What is the profile of a Collapsed Lung patient? While it has been discussed that men are more prone to the condition than women and that a collapsed lung is more probable for those with a tall, lean frame, there is way more to the onset of this condition than meets the eye.

Being one of the one in 1000 women to experience Pneumothorax, Mariska Hartigay has suffered from Collapsed Lung not once, but twice. A top

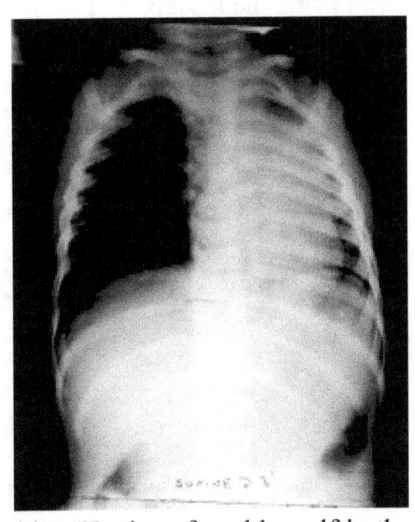

celebrity, with a life full of opportunities, Hartigay found herself in the hospital bed suffering from a sudden attack of Pneumothorax during late October 2008. Otherwise healthy, wealthy and wise, the star was shocked out of her wits when doctors told her that close to 50% of her lungs had collapsed owing to a sharp fall that she took while on the set of the show Law&Order: SVU.

The minute Hartigay landed on the crash pad, she experienced the first symptoms of Pneumothorax; shortness of breath. She says, "*At first I thought I had the wind knocked out of me.*" However, taking it as a simple effect of the fall, she ignored the pain and difficulty in breathing for about three months, after which her condition became unbearable.

After extensive medical treatment and an eventual surgery, Mariska finally recovered after months of rest and no doubt, immense fear. Recalling the time spent at the hospital, she says. "*I had begun to panic, I was so scared... I had so much to lose, so much to live for... I have so many blessings, and I've learned from all of my experiences and my losses.*"

Recalling her mother's death when she was three years old, Mariska reported that her own illness taught her a lot. From just being a celebrity and a mother of a beautiful young boy, she became a person who recognized the bounties of nature and appreciated life for what it was. Today, she is the founder of many charitable organizations, Joyful Heart being the most prominent one that aims to help victims of sexual, domestic and childhood violence.

Causes of Collapsed Lung

If a lung collapse is so dangerous, then how can it be prevented? Or better yet, what measures should be taken to make sure that you are not a victim of this condition? Before these questions can be answered, it is important to understand what causes Pneumothorax. The causes of this ailment have been touched upon briefly in the previous chapter.

Each of these will now be discussed in detail to impart as many facts about Collapsed Lung as possible because this information is crucial for the prevention of the same. In this chapter, the causes of collapsed lungs will be discussed with a wider scope to provide a holistic stance on the subject matter. Once these are understood, classifying each with the type of Pneumothorax under question will be a simple task.

Causes of Injury Related Lung Collapse

As the name suggests, when lungs collapse as a result of an injury, the condition is referred to as Injury Related Lung Collapse. Such collapse is also called Traumatic Pneumothorax as mentioned in the first chapter.

1. Injuries that damage the Chest Cavity:

    Severe injuries that result in damage caused to the chest cavity are the most common cause of Collapsed Lung. A fall or strike that puts excessive pressure in this area or a collision that causes the rib cage to break, can easily result in the leakage of air from the lungs. Once this 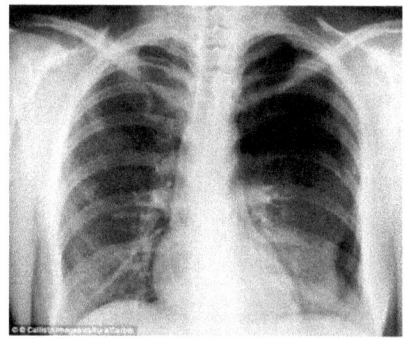 air fills the chest, the patient finds it impossible to breath. A Pneumothorax is most often seen in those who have either been involved in a serious accident or those who end up in a fight with broken bones in the abdominal area.

    Therefore, injuries that result in lung collapse can either be penetrating or non-penetrating.

    Some examples of penetrating injuries include a bullet wound, stabbing, car accidents and falling on sharp concrete surfaces. Non penetrating instances that can result in the same condition are electric shocks, fractured ribs and drowning.

2. Rupture of Air Blisters:

    The appearance and formation of air blebs are quite common among healthy individuals. According to research, these blebs have no reason for their presence along the outer wall of the lungs, nor do they have any purpose or function. Hence, medical experts consider these formations to be harmless; of course, until one or many of the blisters burst and cause air leakage.

While blisters are not associated with a lung disease, if they rupture, a sudden Pneumothorax is the consequence. The rupture can be a result of changes in air pressure, an impact or a collision.

3. Violent Sports:

Violent sport activities like football, rugby and wrestling are some very common causes of lung collapse. Since these sport activities involve a lot of physical contact and are fast paced, a stunt or fall can easily put a lot of added pressure on the lungs, making them tear up. For this reason, sportsmen who suffer from injuries and accidents often end up in the hospital for shortness of breath and due to the inability of the body being able to cope with stress.

Causes of Non-Injury Related Lung Collapse

Non-Injury related lung collapse is the same condition that surfaces even in the absence of an apparent injury. Some common causes of this type include the following:

1. Invasive Surgical Procedures:

   Surgical procedures that involve the use of needles or scalpels are usually performed with the utmost care and sensitivity. The patient, doctors and all those involved in the surgery are, however, aware of the many unprecedented risks that can result from complications and unforeseen circumstances.

   Pneumothorax is one such situation that can arise from invasive surgical procedures. If a needle or any sharp object hits the super sensitive walls of the lungs, a rupture and collapse are an immediate aftermath.

2. Lung Disease:

   Lung Diseases usually damage the lung tissue enough for the organ to stop functioning properly. These diseases result in over worked lungs that do not have the capacity or the strength to provide adequate quantities of oxygen to the body.

   Lung cancer is one such disease that affects millions of Americans each year. It causes lung tissues to inflate, causing damage and making the lungs highly susceptible to tear and collapse because of the weakened walls of this organ.

   Obstructive Pulmonary Disease, Cystic Fibrosis, TB and Pneumonia are some other diseases that severely affect the ability of the lungs to breathe and circulate air normally.

3. Prolonged Ventilation:

   The assistance of a ventilator is often the only way critically ill patients can breathe. When such a patient has become too weak because of chronic illnesses or is brain dead, a ventilator is attached to provide the necessary supply of oxygen and help the lungs deliver it to the other body parts.

When a ventilator pumps air into the lungs, it sometimes causes a lot of pressure to build up. Changes in air pressure can cause the lung walls to tear and collapse. As a result, air leaks into the chest cavity, making the patient breathless with sharp pains in the area. Such a Pneumothorax is usually very severe, affecting the function of the heart as well.

4. Genetics :

    Genetic disorders right from birth are also responsible for causing damage and collapse of the lungs. The Murfan's Syndrome, for instance, is a genetic disorder that degenerates the heart valves. This disease has a direct effect on the lungs and results in frequent lung collapses, often taking the patient's life when combined with other effects.

Coupled with these causes, the risk factors discussed above determine how and when a case of Collapsed Lung is reported. It should be remembered that Primary Spontaneous or Nontraumatic Pneumothorax has no real causes. They occur as a result of normal bodily functions and surprise its victims who are usually very tall and thin males.

Therefore, while the more prominent causes are mentioned above, like lung disease and apparent chest injury, other factors like genetic conditions should also be taken into account when diagnosing a case of Primary Spontaneous Pneumothorax.

How to Know For Sure

How can you be sure that you are a victim of Collapsed Lung? Every time you are short of breath and start coughing, should your senses point to Pneumothorax alone? Accepted that the signs and symptoms of a collapsed lung are hard to pinpoint, especially because they also point to common 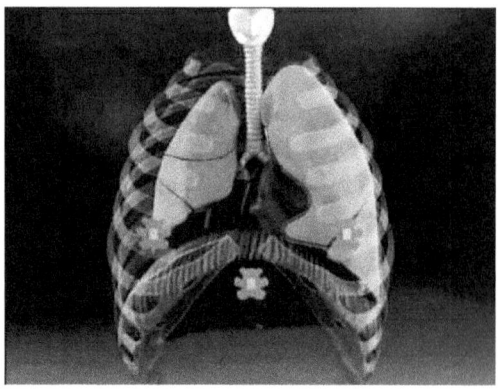 everyday issues, there has to be some guidance regarding the onset of this condition.

Perhaps the biggest problem with Pneumothorax detection is that its causes, signs and symptoms are shared by many other lung injuries and diseases. It is safe to assume that a collapsed lung may be one of the results of continued lung disease. Like in the case of Secondary Spontaneous Pneumothorax, the occurrence of the latter is not always guaranteed because the same signals may well point to another direction.

For instance, Pulmonary Aspiration, a condition that results from the inhalation of salt water, resembles closely to a Collapsed Lung condition because both involve breathlessness, coughing, chest pain and congestion and in extreme cases, unconsciousness. In the aftermath of a Pulmonary Aspiration, a lung tear may never occur; hence, making it quite impossible for you, as a layman, to be quite sure.

Therefore, a proper medical checkup and diagnosis are the best way to decide whether the current situation is a Collapsed Lung case or not. Immediate attention and professional help are the key to preventing a small condition from becoming life threatening. A collapsed lung is usually not fatal to the patient, however, if it is improperly diagnosed, it can cause an increased amount of pressure on the chest cavity and raise the patient's blood pressure and pulse.

It is recommended that you talk to your physician about the signs and symptoms of Pneumothorax beforehand. Knowing what to do in such a condition is the best way to take control of your body and act immediately. Prompt action can help greatly in limiting the damage caused by Collapsed Lung.

Prior knowledge can also help identify this condition should it happen as a case of Primary Spontaneous Pneumothorax. For instance, clinics are increasingly receiving cases of PSP where the young lads, aged between 15 and 20, went through dreadful experiences of sudden lung collapse while they were sleeping or studying for an exam. Being tall and extremely thin, these men are highly prone to PSP from a very young age.

If this information is common among mothers and guardians of young males, it would help them in looking out for a lung collapse attack should they see their child heaving, panting and complaining of even the slightest chest pain. Not only will they then have adequate knowledge about their child's health, they will be mentally prepared to take immediate steps.

Similarly, patients who already have a lung disease should be informed what a Pneumothorax is. While it isn't always necessary that a collapse follows lung disease, should it take after this pattern, the patient will be informed and in a better state of mind to deal with stress.

Symptoms of Collapsed Lung

Most Common Symptoms of Collapsed Lung

Collapsed Lung has many signs and symptoms. Since this condition is related to one of the most crucial and prominent organs of the body, its symptoms are very strong and show as soon as something is amiss. However, because it is a rare condition that isn't at 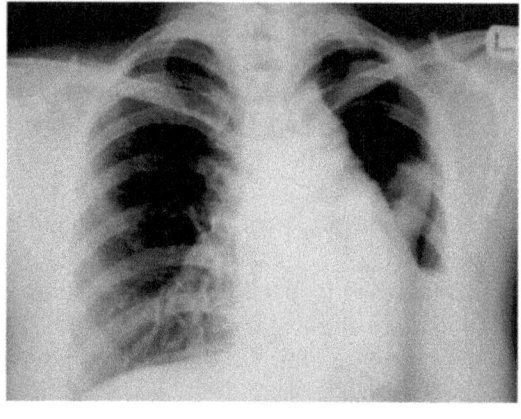 the top of anyone's mind, just like cancer or AIDS would be, the signs of Pneumothorax are often mistaken and ignored.

In the first chapter, we talked about Mariska Hargitay's experience with a collapsed lung that resulted from a sharp fall. Even though she experienced the signs and symptoms of the condition instantly, she ignored them, thinking they were a normal consequence of falling down from a certain height. For three months, she ignored the uneasiness in her chest and the breathing problems she was experiencing until it became unbearable.

Mariska's reaction to the signs of Pneumothorax is not new. Initially, anyone who goes through this condition thinks the symptoms are normal and will pass. However, when the breathing issues continue without any improvement, it becomes apparent that more than just a minor exertion may be the problem.

How can the signs and symptoms of Pneumothorax help in detecting this condition? Doctors advise that as a first step, one needs to become aware of a medical state such as Collapsed Lung because more and more of such cases are being reported nowadays. Awareness regarding this ailment should become more common, so that people know what to do in case its signs are witnessed.

Next, anything that hampers breathing should never be ignored. Even if it is the most insignificant pain experienced while breathing, it should be reported and checked so that immediate action can be taken in case the condition is set to get worse. Thirdly, checking for the signs and symptoms of Pneumothorax at the first stage can make a huge difference to its severity.

For this, however, you need to know what the signs and symptoms of Pneumothorax are. All of these signs are interlinked and one results from the other. Here is a list of the most common ones that you will see in a person after an injury affecting the lungs or when collapse occurs spontaneously.

1. Chest Pains: Sharp and stabbing chest pains are among the first and most aching symptoms of a Pneumothorax. Since air has leaked into the chest cavity, there is a lot of pressure in this area that forces the patient to often lean over and become unstable. When this pain takes over, an individual may feel a similar feeling as that in the case of a heart attack.

    This pain intensifies when the victim tries to breathe, a sensation called Pleuritic.

2. Irritation and constriction of the Abdomen: The entire abdomen feels packed, blocked and constricted. The sensation is similar to the feeling of choking on something because it blocks the windpipe, making it very hard for the patient to breathe normally.

3. Breathlessness: Consequently, breathlessness and a rapid pulse are the result. The pulse may shoot up so high that patients often complain of 'being able to hear their heartbeat.' Breathlessness makes the body very weak and shaky, because of which, one might not be able to move or sit up if collapse occurs during rest or while asleep.

4. Movement of Pain: Unfortunately, the sharp and stabbing pains do not end in the chest cavity. Another very prominent and worrisome symptom of this condition is traveling pain. From

the chest, the pain travels to the neck, shoulders, back and upper arms; gripping the victim in a seizure-like state and making it impossible for them to move or carry on with regular activities.

5. Intense Coughing: The immediate result of breathlessness is coughing. Intense, dry and irritating, such a cough grips the patient, indicating that something is wrong with the lungs and their normal breathing function. Coughing is also a result of a 'filled-up' state of the chest and the pressured position of the diaphragm.

6. Paleness of the face: Doctors have revealed that when Pneumothorax patients arrive in the emergency ward, they are gripping their chest and are pale in the face. Owing to intense coughing and shortness of breath, the color drains from the face, making it yellow. If a Collapsed Lung condition is severe, with an impending cardiac arrest, a patient may appear bluish because of decreased blood flow to the brain and other body parts.

7. Bulging of veins in the neck: Due to increased pressure in the chest cavity, collapsed lungs and shortness of breath, the veins at the nape of the neck bulge out. This indication again points to a severe case of Pneumothorax because constriction in the veins is a signal of a heart attack and increased blood pressure.

8. Shock and Restlessness: Even if the breathlessness is not severe, the patient goes into shock when they feel something blocking their pleural space. Restlessness is very common in cases of minor air leakage because the victim is usually conscious enough to know something is wrong, but in a state of shock to think straight.

9. Loss of consciousness: In extreme cases, mostly in Secondary Spontaneous and Traumatic Pneumothorax, loss of consciousness is also a prominent sign. Because of the lack of oxygen to the brain, the shock and the intense pain, the body succumbs to the pressure and the patient loses consciousness. This sign is not very common among cases of Primary Spontaneous Pneumothorax because the body is otherwise

healthy to stay conscious and fight off the other symptoms mentioned above.

The onset of these signs and symptoms is directly related to how severe the collapse is. If for instance, only a small section of the lung has been affected, only the first three symptoms may be experienced. However, if as much as 50% or more has collapsed, the symptoms will be strong, gripping and often powerful enough to make the patient unconscious.

Early Signs of Collapsed Lung

Whenever you have a serious disease, there is a possibility that you may not recover from it. This is one of the most dangerous situations you can land yourself in. A collapsed lung is one such serious situation and it is important that you recognize the symptoms of this condition at an early stage. After all, you only have one pair of lungs. You have to take exceptional care of them and you have to make sure that you 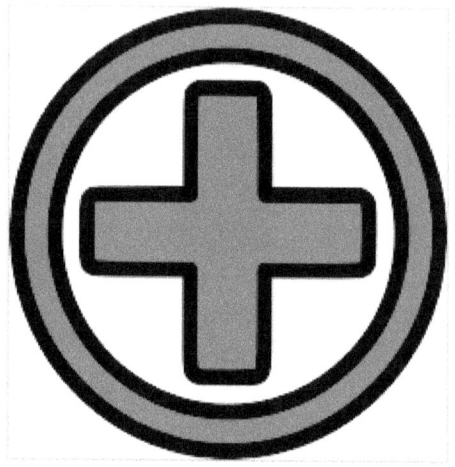 are aware of all signs and symptoms that tell you that your lungs might have collapsed. Here are some signs and symptoms of having a collapsed lung that will help you determine your ailment at an early stage:

- A Sharp Pain In Your Chest:

The first and the biggest red flag that you will encounter when you experience a collapsed lung is a sharp pain in your chest which becomes worse whenever you tend to cough. This pain is centered right where your lungs are situated, which means that it will originate from the middle of your chest and will cause you immense trouble when you sneeze or exert force on them by coughing.

- Respiratory Problems

These respiratory problems are not something that you might get worried about generally. However, minor respiratory problems such as a shortness of breath can also contribute to your diagnosis. You might even experience some difficulty in breathing. These types of minor symptoms usually don't tend to make you anxious and you might attribute them to something else. However, it is in your best interest to not ignore these troubles and see a doctor immediately.

- Fatigue

If your lungs are seriously not working properly, then you can experience fatigue a little too often. Tiring easily is one of the main symptoms of almost any disease. Do not take this ailment lightly because it can be the signal of something very serious. Fatigue is a side effect of 95% of the diseases, so if you are experiencing it, there is no need to act casual about it. Even if it is not a collapsed lung, fatigue can indicate some other illness as well. Be careful and do not ignore it in any way.

- An Increased Pulse

When your lungs collapse, you might end up experiencing a rapid heartbeat which is more serious than it may seem. Heart related diseases, ailments and symptoms are never a good thing since your heart is one of the most important organs of your body. Do not take an increased pulse lightly, no matter what the case, and always refer to a doctor in situations such as these.

- Other Symptoms

There are many symptoms that you will see in yourself if your lungs collapse, and the best way to tell them apart is to see what other symptoms you are experiencing along with the basic ones. Here are a few other symptoms that you will notice in yourself if your lungs are on the verge of collapsing. Tell them apart before it is too late and you will have a chance to avoid a serious setback in your health:

  o Having a bluish skin tone as opposed to your previous skin tone: Blue skin is never really a good sign and when paired with the other basic symptoms of an imminent collapsing lung, it is definitely a sign that should make you worry about your health.

  o Red and Blue spots on the nails are never a good sign: Your nails can forecast and predict a lot of ailments and diseases that your body hasn't caught up to yet. The color of your nails can even predict heart disease before it becomes apparent. In the same way, your nails can tell you if there is something wrong with you before you are past the stage of recovery or of prevention.

- o Flared nostrils while you breathe are known to be another sign that should not be ignored. This one is not as easy to spot but it is another red flag that you should watch out for.

If ever you find yourself experiencing or noticing any one or two of the above mentioned symptoms in your body, you should immediately contact a doctor or a specialist so that he or she can run the specific tests that you need. You will have to get an X-Ray of your lungs to make sure that they are not collapsing. Some other tests might also be in order and these will depend entirely on the physician who will be responsible for your case. Your lungs are not something that you should take for granted; as they say, health is wealth and you should do everything in your power to preserve this wealth as it does not come back once it is gone. Take care of yourself and contact a doctor if these problems occur.

Symptoms for Injury Related Collapsed Lung

Do not remain under the mistaken impression that a collapsed lung cannot occur as result of injury. A lung can collapse due to a number of reasons and one of them can be suffering a great injury to your body. Just as we may experience internal bleeding after receiving trauma to the body, other damages in the body that are not immediately visible include cracked bones, collapsed lungs, concussion and so on. It is very dangerous to move around after suffering a serious injury without getting yourself thoroughly and properly checked by a doctor. Here are a number of ways you can tell that your lungs have collapsed after you have suffered a traumatic and serious injury in the abdominal or chest area of your body:

- Chest Pain

- Lightheadedness

- Trouble Seeing

- Problems with Breathing

- Tightness in the Chest

- Coughing up Blood

Whenever you receive an injury, the signs and symptoms of a collapsed lung are automatically worse than having a non-injury related collapsed lung. An injury tends to aggravate the problem and you can suffer a lot of pain as a result.

The most common cause of injury related Collapsed Lung is a car accident. A car accident, most often than not, causes a severe impact on the torso or the chest. This ends up causing a lot of damage to the organs inside the body; especially the lungs. Even though the lungs and the heart are protected by the ribcage, you can still run a high risk of damaging them. Another possible cause of injury can be when you break a rib and puncture your lung with it. This is one of the most painful experiences anyone can ever face.

The treatment of an injury related collapsed lung is more immediate because it is discovered more easily as compared to a non-injury related collapsed lung. Nevertheless, none of the two are in any way less dangerous than the other.

Symptoms for Non-Injury Related Collapsed Lung

You can have a collapsed lung due to a number of reasons and one of those reasons and one of those reasons is bodily injury. However, injuries are not the sole reason that can cause your lungs to collapse. There are many factors that every physician and every patient need to consider before diagnosing a collapsed lung.

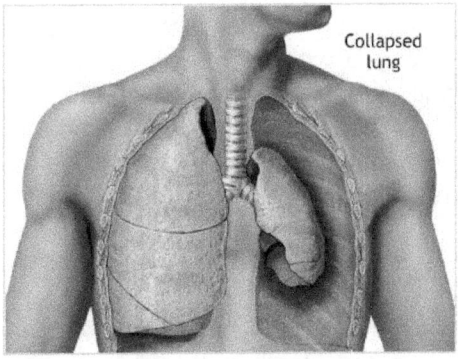

Collapsed lung

Some of these said factors are associated with non-injury related things. Here are a few signs and symptoms that can help you and your diagnostician decide whether you have a collapsed pair of lungs or not:

- Chest Pain

- Shortness of Breath

- Having Trouble Breathing

The above stated symptoms have been discussed in detail in the first section. Here are a number of other symptoms that can help you spot the possibility of a collapsed lung:

- Low Blood Pressure

You might be wondering how you can have an increased pulse but a low blood pressure. This is possible in some patients who do have a collapsed pair of lungs. However, in no patient do all the symptoms become apparent at the same time. In fact, some symptoms occur instead of others, depending on the person's body. So, if you are experiencing low blood pressure do not take it lightly. Blood pressure health related issues are always something serious because your blood pressure is indicating that there is something wrong with the blood circulation mechanism in your body.

- Tightening of the Chest

You might feel some pain and aches in your chest and they will most definitely feel worse when you cough, sneeze or exert too much pressure on your lungs. You will be likely to pass these symptoms off as symptoms of bronchitis or a bad case of the flu or cough. However, what you will not be able to ignore is the tightening of the chest that you might experience when your lungs have collapsed. A constricted chest will make you feel uncomfortable to say the least. It is not something that you can ignore or you might want to experience in the first place.

- Lightheadedness

This is a very common occurrence in people with a collapsed lung. Since the blood in the body is not properly oxygenated due to a collapsed lung, your organs do not get their due share of oxygen. This means that you become lightheaded. This lightheadedness is a clear sign that there is something wrong with your lungs.

Things the Patients Should Remember

As a patient, it is never going to be easy for you at any step of the way. You will experience confusion, pain and even some anxiety, but none of that is even close to how bad things can be if you don't get immediate help. Therefore, during and after your tests you need to be mindful of a handful of things that will help you recover.

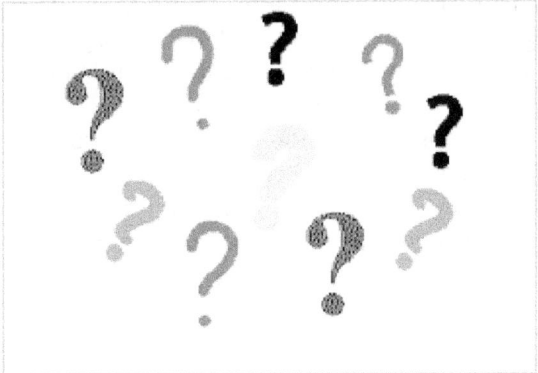

First of all, when you do find out about the problem, then you should not panic or feel anxious. We understand that this is a big health issue and that you might be a little frightened and worried. However, you will get through this if you follow the right steps. The worst thing you can do to yourself is get a panic attack and strain your lungs even further. They need to be relaxed and they need to be tended to immediately. Breathing heavily, becoming anxious or having a panic attack will just make things worse.

You can reduce your anxiety by closing your eyes, sitting in a quiet place and distracting your mind for a while away from this bad news. We know it is going to be hard, but meditation is the best way to get through this period. Even if you were never really good at it, you should keep trying as it is bound to be helpful. Sit down, close your eyes and bring yourself in a state of peace so that your mind gets the message that tension and stress are not the answers to your problem. Rational thought will help you stay calm.

Another tactic would be to start making a list of all the things that can be done. You can start the list with basic and simple points, such as going to see a doctor immediately. Getting treatment and then planning something you have always wanted to do, will be a good way to treat yourself for becoming healthy again. As soon as you start chalking off points, it will bring you closer to your recovery and your brain will start understanding that this problem has a solution and that you are not truly helpless in this situation. This means that you understand the solution and you are only a step away from implementing it in your life. You are not helpless, and this feeling and realization will become your first and most pronounced step towards recovery and towards alleviating the risk of having a panic attack.

There are some things that you need to be concerned about, when you go for your diagnosis. Even though most people will have an understanding attitude regarding your situation, you still do not need to be a difficult patient. As a patient, you should be cooperative and do everything the doctor asks you to do. If you do not listen to the physician and you keep on delaying the diagnosis, then you might suffer the consequences of being diagnosed incorrectly and ending up causing another health problem to yourself.

The doctors who treat you and diagnose you know what they are doing. They have been studying the human body for years and they even have plenty of practical experience treating and diagnosing people with the same condition as you. Leave yourself in their trusted hands and even if you have to bear some pain, take it like a strong patient and do not complain because there is probably no other way your problem can be diagnosed. The experience might be uncomfortable at some points but expect that before you go to the clinic so that you are fully prepared for the diagnostic procedure.

You should also take great care of your hygiene before you go to see a doctor. Take a shower and wash your face and hands properly. If you go to the doctor in filthy attire, yesterday's clothes or smelling bad, it will only make the procedure difficult for both of you. Be clean and look natural so that there are no hindrances when it comes to diagnosing your condition. The doctor will focus on your condition and a lot of makeup might make him miss a few key symptoms that may bring him closer to the right diagnosis of the disease. For example, just as your nails can tell a lot about your health conditions it is best not to cover them in nail paint. Similarly do not use concealer on your dark circles or any pigmentation that might have occurred in a short amount of time in a surprising manner. Anything in your appearance that may seem out of the ordinary should be told to the doctor so that they can note that down and draw a conclusion.

You should bear in mind that the tests and the physical examination might become uncomfortable at some point but before anything makes you so, the doctor will exclusively tell you that "this might feel a little odd" or "this can get a little painful or uncomfortable" so that you are prepared for whatever comes next.

Here are a number of tips and tricks that will help you get through the tough times:

- Do not talk in a loud voice or exert a lot of force on your lungs

- Take lots of rest and try not to speak needlessly. Only speak when it is necessary.

- Follow the treatment that your doctor or physician instructs you to do. Do not use your own knowledge and do not make any modifications. If you have questions, do not be afraid to ask your doctor.

- Whenever you cough a lot, take some cough drops to refrain from putting a lot of strain on your lungs.

- Try not to laugh a lot, especially with a lot of force. Do not resort to the kind of laughter that 'leaves you in stitches'.

- Do not, under any circumstances, smoke a cigarette or consume alcohol or drugs.

- Ask questions and stay up to date with your treatment procedures. Be aware of your recovery timeline as well.

- Make sure that you know what activities you are allowed to indulge in and what activities you should be giving up (especially at the moment).

- Make sure you know how to take care of your own self.

- Are there any problems that you need to watch out for? Ask the doctor what to do if something goes awry.

- Stay updated and come back for regular checkups.

- If the pain is a little extreme, you can take pain killers but don't make a habit of this. You can also prop up a handful of pillows whenever you face any kind of trouble breathing so that you can assist your lungs in all the ways that you can.

In the end, whatever the result may be, hold your head high and stay strong. Do not cave into depression and do not give up because you can fight this problem, It is not incurable. You just have to stay strong and not give in to any anxiety that you may end up feeling.

Treatment for Collapsed Lung

Stages of Collapsed Lung

Having a collapsed lung is nothing to be taken lightly and like any other ailment, there are several stages of suffering and eventually recovering from a collapsed lung. These stages help us determine what part of the ailment we are currently facing and what we can then do to make the treatment more effective. As a patient 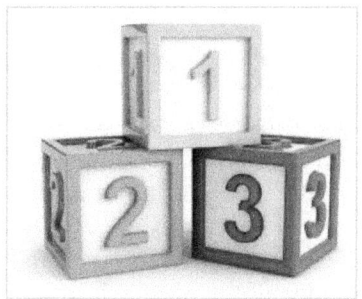 you have to understand that your entire experience will be, and this iscalculated in three stages:

- **Diagnosis – The Initial Stage**

The Diagnosis stage comes after you recognize the symptoms of a collapsed lung. Recognizing and pin pointing the signs and symptoms is one of the most important stages that will help you get to the second and then all the way to the final stage. In the initial stages, you will experience symptoms such as chest pain, breathing problems, tightness in the chest and even lightheadedness or fatigue. However, if you have a collapsed lung because of an injury or an accident, then you will see that you might even cough up blood. This entirely depends upon the type and the seriousness of the injury that you have sustained. When you are getting diagnosed, you will require a lot of courage and levelheadedness. You have to be strong and take the situation head on. You have to visit the doctor and confide in him regarding the signs and symptoms that you are experiencing or have been experiencing for a while. Then the doctor will conduct some tests, ask you questions and then tell you what you are suffering from. The diagnosis helps determine the treatment of the condition you are suffering from.

- **Treatment – The Second Stage**

This stage is all about fighting the problem and sticking with the treatment routine that your doctor has advised. You have to be on time, do not miss any appointments and always follow up with checkups.

Your treatment will take some time and it is imperative that you ask questions and keep yourself up to date with the entire situation. Abstain from things that the doctor tells you to stay away from and do not indulge in strenuous and exerting activities. The treatment will take some time but if you do what the doctor tells you then you will find yourself recovering in no time.

- **Post – Treatment – The Final Stage**

The recovery stage is very important because this is where you have to exercise great caution. If you were a smoker in the past, then you have to quit smoking now because it is not good for your lungs. You also have to abstain from very strenuous exercise so as not to exert a lot of pressure on your recovering lungs. You have to eat wisely and then follow all the dietary instructions that your doctor has given you. Keep on meeting with your doctor to find out how the recovery process is going. Treating a collapsed lung is not half as tough and complicated as the recovery stage, so you have to be very careful. Don't lose focus and become careless in any way.

When to Seek Medical Attention

"When should I seek medical attention?" This question is on the mind of every individual who suffers from any kind of illness or ailment. No matter what type of disease or ailment they are suffering from, people are always unsure about what they are supposed to do, how they are supposed to cope with it and when they should seek help from a doctor. Many people are a little scared of going to the doctor and discovering they might have something that is very dangerous, while others believe that the symptoms are nothing but minor allergies or small illnesses. This allows them to ignore their symptoms and 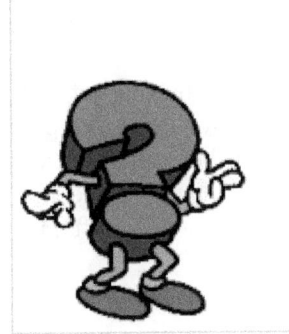 their illness until it is too late for them. However, you should not be so cavalier about your health and you should go see a doctor immediately even if you are a little unsure about the symptoms you are noticing and experiencing in your body.

Here are a few symptoms that should prompt you to visit and consult a doctor at a moment's notice. You should not delay this as it can end up causing you a lot of damage if things get out of hand.

- The first red flag for you should be the chest pain that you might start experiencing at the start. This chest pain could be there for a variety of reasons but it is mostly never anything that you should ignore or not pay any heed to. Most times, chest pain is very dangerous and it speaks of even more dangerous health ailments. Do not take it lightly in any way.

- When you experience any blunt trauma to your lungs which can hurt your ribs or your lungs in any way, e.g. If you fall on your chest or if someone punches you in the torso it is always a good idea to meet with the doctor and see if there is any damage.

- When you start coughing up blood especially after a blunt trauma to the chest or torso or even after a small injury. Coughing up blood, also known as hemoptysis, is never ever a good sign for anyone.

- Respiratory problems are the next and last symptom that you need to notice before you consider consulting a doctor about this. Do not wait for other small and less frequent symptoms to appear, because by the time that will happen, it will probably be too late. Rely on your instincts and contact the doctor when you experience chest pain or other respiratory problems such as shortness of breath and trouble breathing.

Even if you suspect that it is not a collapsed lung, when you experience the above listed symptoms, you should most definitely drop in to see a doctor because these signs could predict a much more serious illness or injury that may be hidden at the moment. Do not take your health casually – it's a gift and you should treasure it!

Common Treatments

Over the years, as the causes and occurrence of Pneumothorax become clearer, various treatment options have been devised. While the condition itself is not fatal, if left undetected for too long, a collapsed lung can have disastrous side effects – most of which begin with added stress on the heart. All treatment options aim to restore the form, shape, size and functionality of the lungs so that oxygen is delivered to the body just as normal.

Moreover, the treatments available to deal with Collapsed Lung also aim to bring the pressure of air back to normal in the chest cavity. When this pressure is out of balance, the chest feels constricted and breathing becomes problematic. Therefore, prompt treatment of Pneumothorax is not only necessary, it is the best way to ensure that the damage does not reach the heart.

However, do all types of Pneumothorax need treating?

Conservative Treatment

Mild lung collapses, in which only a small portion of the organ is affected- less than 30%- do not need invasive treatment. Diagnosis for such a condition is done in the same manner, using X-Rays and CT Scans and consultations with experts. Many doctors put victims of minor collapses under observation to see how well the lungs are coping and whether penetrative measures are needed. An external oxygen supply may be the only treatment necessary in this instance.

There have been many cases of Pneumothorax in which the small amount of air that had leaked into the chest cavity escapes on its own, letting the lung come back to its original shape and size. If this is the case, ample rest and some painkillers are prescribed. Patients are told to allow their body to recuperate from the attack. According to evidence, it can take close to 3-6 weeks for the collapse to heal completely, after which, these patients can carry on normal activities.

Such a treatment option is called "Conservative Treatment". Since the chances of respiratory failure are very low, doctors prefer to let the body take care of the abnormality, albeit, under strict observation. If symptoms seem to normalize, patients are also allowed to go home with instructions to report back immediately should the condition escalate.

Aspiration & Chest Tube Treatment

If a Pneumothorax affects 50% or more of the lungs, Conservative Treatment is not enough. Such a case is usually characterized by extreme breathlessness and the patient's body is unable to cope with the stress. When it is apparent that an invasive treatment is the only solution, doctors usually use two treatment options. These are:

1. Aspiration – Aspiration is the removal of an air rim from the space between the ribs. In other words, air is sucked out of the pleural space so that the lungs can inflate again and the added pressure on the organs can be stabilized. Aspiration involves the insertion of a needle into the chest cavity, after local anesthesia is administered. This needle is connected to a three way tap through which air is allowed to escape when the doctor initiates suction. A volume of 2.5 liters can be drawn out via aspiration, making this one of the most effective and moderately invasive ways to treat a collapsed lung. After this volume, the remaining air is allowed to escape on its own and the patient is kept under observation.

   More than 50% of mild-major cases of Pneumothorax are treated with the insertion of a needle to suck out the collected air. This method is most used in PSP cases because the lack of a complicated medical history means the patient is strong enough to bear this procedure.

2. Chest Tube- The second, more intrusive yet definitive method of air withdrawal is inserting a chest tube into the body. Pneumothorax cases that are likely to recur with a superficial aspiration are treated with a chest tube so that the condition can be cured for good. The chest tube is inserted from the side, under the armpit, so that it does not come in the way of other organs of the body.

   Even though this process can be completed under local anesthesia, a lot of care should be exercised because of its invasive nature. Once inserted, the tube draws out air via a one-way valve. The size of the chest tubes used depends on the extent of the Pneumothorax in question.

Regular observation and monitoring are key to the success of this treatment. X-rays are performed at intervals to keep an eye on the size of the air rim. When no more air seems to be escaping the chest cavity over a period of time, a final X-ray is done to gauge progress. Chest Tube Insertion is the best way to treat SSP because in the presence of other complications, a quick solution to a collapse is needed.

If, 2–4 days pass and progress is limited, this may be an indication that the Chest Tube Treatment is ineffective for a particular case. In this scenario, surgery is the most appropriate option.

Surgical Treatment

Surgical Treatment, though highly penetrative, is the only solution to long term and recurring Pneumothorax. Medically called Pleurodesis, surgery for a collapsed lung involves the permanent obliteration of the pleural space. This means that the cavity in which air has collected will be reduced as much as possible.

Pleurodesis is a two-step process. Through a large incision in the middle of the chest, the surgeon first stitches up any tears found along the outer walls of the lungs or staples the blebs that have ruptured. Once this source of leakage is taken care of, the lungs are then stitched to the chest wall to help the patient breath better, with no risk of the pleural space being filled up.

The recurrence rate after Pleurodesis is as low as 1%, making this surgery highly effective. Another variation of Pleurodesis is often practiced by surgeons when there is an option to keep the pleural space intact. When no rupture or tear is in sight, instead of sewing the lungs to the chest walls, the surgeon sprays a talc like powder all over the exposed organ. This powder acts like an irritant that inflames the lungs and then sticks to them to heal any ruptures that are invisible to the naked eye. This way, the pleural space is not obliterated, making the procedure less intensive.

Conclusion

The treatments discussed here are diverse in scope and nature. In the presence of such innovative and evolutionary treatment options, Pneumothorax has become a manageable condition. The effort that goes into its detection is well compensated for by the array of options that are available in the field of Pulmonary Medicine to diagnose and treat all stages of Pneumothorax.

Who can treat it?

The signs, symptoms, causes, reactions and results of a Pneumothorax all indicate that this condition shouldn't be taken lightly. While a collapsed lung isn't fatal, the reasons for its occurrence are often unclear and vague, making doctors and health care professionals all the more concerned about it.

The previous discussion about the treatment methods of Pneumothorax details the ways in which the lungs should be treated in varying cases and severity levels. These treatments have been developed over the years, as more information has been revealed via extensive studies and better technology has become available.

However, it is undeniable that treatments are as good as the person performing them. While any doctor can prescribe a painkiller, not every professional can give the best service when it comes to treating a condition with needles, chest tubes and CT Scans. Since the procedures to treat a ruptured or collapsed lung are highly technical, they require the doctor to be very skilled and experienced.

Think about the following instances:

- If the chest tube is inserted incorrectly, the Pneumothorax can worsen to a greater degree, so much so that it can turn into a fatal ailment. Inability to breath, sudden shock and an increase in blood pressure can result from the incorrect administration of corrective measures.

- If the needles for aspiration are not inserted with caution, they can result in more ruptures and even a tear in the lung that may not have been present initially.

- If, during surgery, the sutures on the lungs are not properly sterilized, they can result in the spread of infection throughout the body.

- Unavailability of CT scan machines can lead to incomplete diagnosis of the condition, in which case there are no grounds to treat it properly.

- Lack of staff in ER may leave you in a critical state of breathlessness, escalating the collapsed condition even more.

- Unhygienic conditions that raise questions about the sterilization of needles can lead to many diseases and viruses within the premises of the health care facility.

Hence, there is no question that Pneumothorax should only be treated at fully functional hospitals and private clinics that have all equipment in place and are attended by some of the most skilled and professional medical experts. Advanced procedures such as these should only be performed by a Pulmonologist who is an expert in every kind of lung and respiratory disease.

However, not every hospital has a Pulmonologist on the panel. In the absence of one, Pneumothorax cases are handled by General Surgeons who take advice from other colleagues if a complicated case is under question. Nonetheless, to make sure you are seeing the best of doctors, especially if you already have underlying lung disease, always ask for a Pulmonologist to overlook your medical case.

Moreover, if a local or neighborhood clinic lacks the necessary equipment like needles and chest tubes, it is best to avoid going to such a facility. Similarly, improper staffing is another problem that many hospitals face nowadays. Only one doctor attending an ER that is full of patients is a sign that the hospital/clinic is not managed properly.

Apart from these main concerns, taking note of the hygiene and general working of the facility is also imperative because you and your loved ones are the only people who can ensure you get the best attention, treatment and care for your body. Therefore, always make sure to go to medical centers that are known for and specialize in Pulmonology Diseases and Remedies.

Prevention

How to Prevent Collapsed Lung

Even though a condition like Pneumothorax is not fatal in its initial stages (a very low death rate has been reported) those who learn about it are always interested to know how to prevent it from happening. A concerned mother of a 15 year old, tall and thin boy will definitely be on the lookout for prevention tips to make sure she can help her child in any way possible.

Therefore, discussing the prevention of Collapsed Lung is important. Since this condition is highly painful, with signs and symptoms that can rob an individual of performing everyday tasks, knowing how to prevent its occurrence is a good way to look after your health. The prevention of Collapsed Lung is best studied and implemented when one takes into account the various types of Collapsed Lung that patients are diagnosed with.

Prevention of Various Types of Pneumothorax

Injury Related Collapse

In the case of Injury Related Pneumothorax, not much can be done to ensure the safety of the lungs. If the chest cavity has been crushed, stabbed or penetrated, the lungs are likely to be damaged in the process. Hence, Traumatic Lung Collapse is often unavoidable if the accident or injury is severe.

Therefore, first of all, if you know about collapsed lungs being a result of most chest-related accidents, be careful. Do not take part in fights, especially those that can get rough. Try your best to avoid getting injured in the abdominal area because damage to the lungs and consequently, the heart, is sustained easily.

Another way a Traumatic Lung Collapse can be avoided is when the trauma is tended to immediately. Getting a doctor's help as soon as you get hurt is crucial to limit the damage to the body.

Injury Related Lung Collapse can also occur in contact sports. Violent sports activities like wrestling, football, weight lifting and rugby can damage the chest cavity and weaken the walls of the lungs easily. Sportsmen who would do anything to win are often advised by their physicians to take it slow and look after their bodies over and above the desire of a win.

Prevention of a lung collapse due to such sports activities can be done *via* the following ways:

- Getting a full and detailed checkup before taking part in violent sports.

- Understanding the rules and limits of the sport properly to avoid getting hurt unnecessarily. Following these rules should never be an option.

- Giving your body the importance it deserves, even if that means losing a game.

- If a casual sport has a high injury rate, it is best to avoid it. Basing this decision on adrenaline and excitement alone is not right. For instance, bungee jumping is an attractive sports activity undertaken by those with a desire for adventure. Since it involves risking your life while jumping from a high altitude, an adverse effect on the body, particularly the lungs, is hard to avoid owing to the changes in air pressure through the fall. When the lungs are exposed to the varying degrees of pressure, tissue damage and leakage of air are likely results.

  Therefore, sportsmen who consider this activity casual fun should be very cautious before doing so because it can result in a Pneumothorax instantly.

Non-Injury Related Collapse

The second type of Lung Collapse is Non-Injury Related. Injury related lung collapse could be controlled by limiting the extent of injury, but how can Non-Injury Related Collapse be avoided? What Prevention tips can you keep in mind at all times? Moreover, is prevention even possible?

Non-Injury Related Pneumothorax is further divided into Primary and Secondary Lung Collapse. Both these conditions have different stimuli and are controlled in varying ways. In the case of Primary Spontaneous Pneumothorax, the victim is taken by surprise as they are otherwise a healthy individual. Due to the nature of the attack, it makes it quite impossible for people to prevent it.

If your son is healthy and away at college, it wouldn't even be in your wildest imagination that his lung could collapse while sleeping. Such has been the situation for many guardians who couldn't understand why their child was the victim of this ailment. As mentioned previously, the child's physique should raise alarm bells for parents who have young boys in the 15 to 20 age bracket.

PSP can be prevented when parents talk to their child about the possibility of this ailment and what to do if it happens. The following tips should be discussed with them.

- Avoid smoking because it weakens the walls of the lungs. Youngsters can fall into the pattern of smoking and drug abuse. Make sure your child is well aware of the adverse effects of these habits.

- If your son is going through sudden growth spurts, get regular appointments with the doctor for general checkups. Ask the doctor for tips on how to avoid any lung related problems all throughout the growth period.

- Sometimes, a lung collapse occurs because of constant exposure to harsh environments that are saturated with chemical fumes or other harmful substances. Try to avoid such conditions as much as possible.

- If your child has gone through PSP once, there is a 25% chance of recurrence. To prevent this, follow your doctor's advice as much as possible, keep them away from varying air pressure zones and take care of the wounds (in case of surgery) by attending regular follow-ups.

Secondary Spontaneous Pneumothorax is the result of an underlying lung disease. This type of collapse is most common in men over 40 years of age. Tips to ensure prevention are:

- Avoid smoking at all costs.

- It is preferable for you to avoid air travel if you have lung disease because the possibility of a Pneumothorax is much higher than a regular person.

- Discuss the possibility of this condition with your doctor. If advised, prior action can be taken to prevent it altogether.

- Take the lung disease medication strictly on time, so the condition doesn't get worse, leading to a collapse of the lungs.

- Avoid undue stress. Stress releases certain hormones in the body, the excess of which can result in lung tissue damage.

Diagnosis

Most Common Diagnosis for Collapsed Lung

Like any other ailment, Pneumothorax has a standard diagnostic procedure that is followed by medical professionals every time such a case is brought to a hospital or clinic. Even though it is often hard to be sure whether the condition under question is Pneumothorax, once the diagnosis is performed, a clearer picture can be generated.

If you look at an individual who is panting, clutching their chest and looking very pale, can you immediately say they are suffering from Collapsed Lung? No. Since air leakage needs to be investigated thoroughly before a conclusion can be drawn, a series of steps need to be followed before, during and after diagnosis, for a Pneumothorax case to be treated accordingly.

Important Steps for Diagnosis and Post-Diagnosis

Diagnosis of Pneumothorax is completed *via* the following steps. These steps are somewhat the same for every kind of Pneumothorax, but are specific to PSP because in the case of SPS and Injury Related Lung Collapse, the protocol is much more strict and swift.

1. Rush to the ER- Be it a severe case of Lung Collapse or a minor one, the victim should immediately be taken to the ER of the closest hospital or clinic. For the diagnosis to begin and the treatment to be given, going to a medical facility is a must because Pneumothorax requires proper care and attention. If the air leakage is very small in quantity, the symptoms may pass in a few minutes. However, getting a thorough checkup is still the most advisable course of action.

2. Explain your condition to a doctor in the ER- When you are at the ER and a doctor is tending to you, the first question you will be asked is regarding the pain you felt, its severity and other

symptoms you have experienced in the last few minutes or hours. Explaining your health condition to the doctor honestly is very important for a detailed and accurate diagnosis.

3. Examination- The next step is examination. Once you have told the attending doctor how you feel and the symptoms you have experienced, they will do a thorough checkup. This includes, taking your pulse, listening to the heart, and checking your breathing and blood pressure using a stethoscope. The amount of pain you have also determines how sharp or dull your reflexes have become. All of these measurements are part of the preliminary exam.

4. Tests- From the results of the preliminary exam and the continuation of signs and symptoms like coughing, breathlessness and becoming pale in color, the doctor will order for some tests to be done. These tests will reveal the inner condition of the body, i.e. whether there is a tear in the lung, if the chest cavity has been injured or if ruptured blisters can be detected.

The most commonly conducted tests for Pneumothorax include MRI, Ultrasound, X-rays and CT Scans. All of these methods are used to get cross-sectional views of the abdominal area so that a 3D image of the lungs can be studied for conclusions.

- X-ray: Diagnosis of any type of lung collapse starts with an X-ray or radiograph of the chest. Patients who have suffered a Pneumothorax are radiographed from the back because this position yields the best images of the condition of the lungs. Side by side, lateral X-Rays are also taken so that a complete picture of the lungs is taken before any conclusions are drawn.

  A good X-ray examined by a professional can help determine the size of the Pneumothorax. This is done by measuring the distance between the chest wall and the lungs. If this distance is abnormal, it is safe to assume that air has filled up in the cavity. Since all Pneumothorax's are different in size and nature, an accurate diagnosis is the key to treating this condition effectively.

Many times, an X-ray fails to show a Pneumothorax. However, if the doctors strongly suspect its existence, other methods are used to aid the radiograph.

- CT scan: A CT Scan is a very useful diagnostic tool because it helps doctors identify whether the abnormality in the chest cavity is a Pneumothorax or just an enlarged bullae. The CT scan is superior to an X-ray because if a patient cannot sit upright for a radiology film, the appearance of a collapse may not be very clear. In this situation, a CT scan helps to get 3D imagery that is detailed and dissected such that every part of the lungs can be examined.

- Ultrasound: An ultrasound is a sensitive test that can detect the smallest Pneumothorax. This diagnostic tool is used in cases where the patient has gone through a traumatic injury and the chest has been penetrated. Determining the size of the collapse is not only easy with an ultrasound, it is also the quickest way to come to a conclusion in an emergency.

5. Consultation: Once the test results are received, the actual diagnosis can be made. Studying these results, together with the patient's medical history and the way they are holding up, doctors make conclusions regarding the severity of the attack. The space in the chest cavity that is occupied by air, any damage to the lungs and the state of the heart are all visible when these scans are done. To come to a conclusion regarding the plan of action, doctors usually consult each other and arrive at a unanimous decision regarding how the patient should be treated.

6. Preparing For Surgery/Procedure- If the doctors decide that the Pneumothorax is significant and surgery is needed, you will be prepared for one. Surgery in this case is not very complicated; however, adequate preparation is still needed, and since breathing is difficult with a lung collapse, the doctors will prioritize your surgery over others that can wait.

On the other hand, if the collapse is minor, you may be admitted to the hospital/clinic for a chest syringe procedure that is done under local anesthesia to remove air from the chest cavity.

7. Surgery/Procedure- The actual surgery or procedure is then performed. This may take anywhere between 2 to 5 hours in total, depending on the procedures, need for preparation and the actual surgery time. Generally a chest syringe procedure is easier and simpler than sewing up a tear on the side of the lungs.

8. Recovery- Recovery is the last step in which the lungs are allowed to heal and recover. Because of excessive panting, breathlessness and pain, the body will need ample time and rest to recover fully. A period of at least 10 days is needed for even those who do not have any prior lung conditions to start with.

What Works?

When you are diagnosed with a collapsed lung, the last thing you should be doing is losing hope and panicking. There is nothing worse than a low morale and giving up before the fight has even started. Many people tend to get discouraged and lose hope even before they have the chance to recover. This is why when you get diagnosed with Collapsed Lung the first thing you have to tell yourself is that it is curable and it will be treated by doctors if you maintain the right attitude along the way. You need to focus on what can heal you instead of all those things that have the potential to destroy you.

Since the excess air or fluid in your lungs is harming you, the doctor will probably put a tube in your lungs to drain the fluids and to remove excess air from your lungs. If it is a very minor and unnoticeable problem then they might not pay a lot of attention to it; however, if they see that it is becoming something harmful they will definitely try to insert the tube in your lungs. Extra blood is also removed from the lungs so that they can function in a proper manner. The doctors will also ensure that the lungs in your body stay out of harm's way when they are being treated. This precaution is to ensure that your lungs do not get side-tracked during the healing process.

Since your body is being treated, you become even more vulnerable to other diseases that might be just as dangerous for you. This can result in greater problems. The doctors will treat you and take care of you as you recover so that a greater and graver problem can be avoided before it occurs. The tube that is inserted into your lungs does the job of draining unwanted substances out of your lungs and it also ensures that no other unwanted substances find their way back into your lungs again. Since your lungs will be weak when you treat them, they need some extra protection and precautionary measures whilst you are treating them. You are not born with an extra pair of lungs, so you need to take care of the ones that you have.

Medication and Procedures

Whenever you get diagnosed for a particular disease, your first course of action is to find out what can help you recover from the disease. You will most likely find a doctor who will be able to treat you. Then you will find out what procedures can help treat your disease or your condition. In addition to that, the doctor will also prescribe a number of medicines that will not only help you heal, but will also protect you through the entire process of treatment.

For most people, the mere thought of treatment can prove to be a frightful concept. They fear that the treatment will bring with it a lot of pain, inconvenience and plenty of other complications or side effects. The idea that medication does more damage than good has been instilled in every single person's mind. This has caused a lot of unnecessary panic among many patients who are seeking treatment to recover from a particular disease or ailment.

The Treatment Procedure

If you have a collapsed lung, the first thing that you have to do is look for a capable doctor who knows what to do and how to treat you. When you have found a doctor who will properly be able to treat you, you need to understand what procedure will be used to cure your ailment. This is because you need to be aware of all the things you need to do to facilitate the process. If you are unaware of what the procedure is, you are bound to do something that might end up harming you even more. If you have all the knowledge and are aware of all the facts, then it becomes easier for you to recover.

There are several ways of treating Collapsed Lung but the treatment procedure is basically determined using the information regarding your disease or ailment. The doctor first figures out how much damage has been inflicted on your lungs, how badly you have been afflicted with the condition and at what stage of the disease you are facing at the moment. When all of this information has been procured and the basic things have been determined, the doctor proceeds with the treatment. The most popular form of treatment is draining the liquid or blood out of the lungs.

When you have water, blood or extra air in your lungs, the doctors can insert a tube in the lungs and then drain out all of the liquid or extra air from them, so that they can come back to their healthy state. This is a simple yet very important procedure that can make you healthy once more.

The Medication

There are many medicines that are involved in the treatment of Collapsed Lung. Just as with every major disease or ailment, the treatment requires you to be on plenty of medication. Here are a number of medicines that your doctor might prescribe during your treatment so that you can recover faster and better: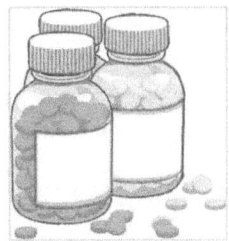

- *Pain Medication*

Pain medication is a given in diseases and ailments such as these. In most, if not all cases, the pain medication (no matter how strong it is) does not relieve 100% of the pain. There is always that small tinge of pain or discomfort the person still experiences. The basic purpose of pain medication is to reduce the pain to a level that allows you to carry out your day to day activities.

Basic pain medication only caters to short term pain as it has not been designed keeping in mind the specific details of long term pain or chronic pain. Most of the time, when people go to the hospital, they are prescribed pain medication that is only sufficient until the next checkup. If the follow-up is delayed then the painkiller will not be good enough.

Extensive and careless use of pain medication can cause a lot of unnecessary problems and dangerous complications. This is one of the reasons why the trauma centre does not refill pain medication over the phone and does not give you an extra supply of painkillers to last for a few more days.

- *Opioid Medication*

Opioid medications help alter the way the brain perceives or processes the element of pain. However, they can prove to be rather dangerous if not administered properly to the patient. When you take Opioid medication you should be careful regarding the following points:

- o Do not consume alcohol

- o Do not do drugs

- o Do not share them with anyone

- o Do not prolong the use of Opioid medication

- o If possible, take the smallest dose

- o When you are on the medication it would be best for you not to drive a car

- o When you are on the medication it would be best for you not to operate heavy machinery.

- o When you are on the medication it would be best for you not to be responsible for the care of other people.

- o Do not consume sleeping pills, anxiety pills or any other such medication

- o Get rid of Opioid medication once you are done with it by driving it to the drug collection site.

- o Be mindful of all the side effects of Opioid Medication. The side effects can range from constipation to decreased breathing whilst sleeping. Even though constipation is the less dangerous side effect you must do everything in your power to make it easier on you. You must consume a lot of water, and whenever necessary opt for a laxative. If you have decreased breathing while sleeping at night, note that it can prove to be very deadly. You need to be more careful about this side effect and get medical help because it can end up taking your life. Ask your friends and family to watch out for you when or if that happens to you in your sleep, since you will be unaware of it yourself.

When you are looking for a treatment for Collapsed Lung you have to make sure that you have a proper doctor who understands your situation. The effectiveness of the medication is the secondary factor in this case. This is because the most important thing is to have a good doctor by your side who can guide you through all these things. Even if you do have good medicines, you will not fully recover until and unless your doctor treats you properly. If the doctor misunderstands your body and your condition then the quality of the procedure, the work and the medicines take a backseat.

In this case, if the doctor understands your body and prescribes it what it needs instead of prescribing it the standard things, you will be able to recover in a faster, better and happier manner than other people who do not have great doctors. When you search for a doctor make sure that you have made the right choice because it can end up making or breaking your life.

Living With Collapsed Lungs

Day to Day Activities

Many patients who have been diagnosed with Collapsed Lung find it hard adjusting to ordinary day to day life. This is because many things that healthy people take for granted and assume to be no problem at all cause a lot of complications, dangers and problems for people who have been diagnosed with a collapsed lung.

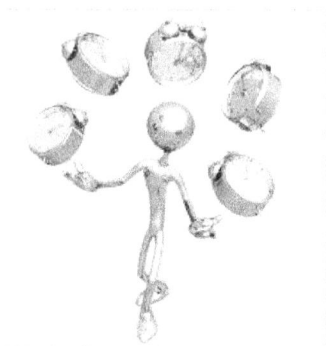

Most patients who have been diagnosed with a collapsed lung are allowed to resume their daily activities when they go to a doctor. The doctor advises them not to halt their tasks and mess up their daily routine, or allow the ailment to get the better of them. Counter-intuitively, the patient is advised to carry on with their life regardless of the disease he or she is inflicted with.

There are many things that can help you on your road to recovery and all of those things have been mentioned here so that you can better acquaint yourself with them. Almost half of the patients who have a collapsed lung face a recurrence and you should do everything in your power to make sure that you do not face that. Here are a number of things you should do to make sure you can keep up with your ordinary day to day activities and still maintain a normal life:

Go On With Your Life Regardless of Your Ailment

Carrying on with daily life activities is important for a patient because this way, the disease or the ailment does not take over the life of the patient completely. If the patient lets the disease affect every single facet of his or her life and starts thinking that they cannot do anything because they have an ailment, they will cage themselves in the disease and possibly become even sicker. However, if the person goes on with their daily routine and does not let the disease cripple them in any way, they have a better chance of fighting it off than someone who becomes their disease.

Do not Laugh Out Loud

There is nothing wrong with a little light laughter but you should refrain from the kind of laughter that gives you a stomach ache, makes it harder to breathe or brings tears to your eyes. A healthy pair of lungs can handle something like that. A collapsed lung, on the other hand, is a completely different story when it comes to laughing uncontrollably.

Even with a healthy pair of lungs, some people find it hard to breathe when they are laughing. Imagine what would happen if someone with a collapsed lung started laughing uncontrollably and found himself or herself completely unable to breathe. You can only assume how bad it could actually get.

Refrain from Strenuous exercise

If you have a collapsed lung, strenuous and heavy exercise can prove to be very dangerous for you. When you are jogging or running you often find yourself out of breath. You also probably know of the significance of inhaling and exhaling deeply when it comes to working out strenuously at the gym or at home. When you inhale and exhale, you have to do these with a lot of energy and you can imagine how much strain this puts on your lungs. While a healthy pair of lungs would have no problem dealing with that kind of stress, if you have a collapsed lung then you might find yourself in a very dangerous situation if you put your lungs under stress.

Cooking

You have to be a little careful when you are making something over the stove. When you are cooking you generally stand near the stove and take in all the smells and aromas that waft up from the stove. The food being cooked is placed on a fire, which is why at some point the food also produces smoke. This smoke is not as thick as some you see in bonfires or in camp fires, but the smoke is still relatively thicker than the air around it. This means that your lungs will be inhaling some amount of extra moisture from the air when you are cooking, in addition to all the extra substances in the smo ke wafting up from the meal.

Helping Aids for People with Collapsed Lungs: First Aid

When you want to live your daily life despite the fact that you have a collapsed lung, you have to understand that from time to time you will require a few helping aids. There may be times when you feel perfectly fine going about day to day work but then there are times when you do not know how to even handle the situation. You need to adapt to the situation and understand as much as you can about your condition. In addition to that, you and your friends should also be well aware of how to administer first aid in case of emergencies so that the damage can be minimized instead of being aggravated due to the wrong kind of first aid being administered in time of emergencies.

Administering First Aid to a Patient with Collapsed Lung

In the life of a person who is dealing with Collapsed Lung, there may come some instances where they might find themselves unable to breathe. In these conditions, the friend or family member present at the scene needs to administer flawless first aid. Here is how to help a person breathe in such a time of distress:

- Step 1: If you know CPR then you must first administer that to your friend who is finding himself or herself unable to breathe. You need to check the person's breathing, his or her pulse and his or her airways.

- Step 2: Loosen any tight clothing he or she might be wearing at the time. Tight clothing can be very dangerous as it can end up constricting the airways and making the situation even more complicated and dangerous for the patient.

- Step 3: Call for medical assistance because no matter how good you are with CPR, it will only hold you off for a short while. After that the patient may have trouble breathing once again. Always ask someone to call for medical assistance or call for it yourself because you cannot take the huge risk of neglecting such a situation.

- Step 4: You must monitor the person's breathing and the breathing patterns he or she has at that moment. Also be sure to check and monitor the person's pulse very carefully until medical assistance arrives. Even if wheezing or abnormal breathing sounds and abnormal breathing patterns cannot be spotted anymore, do not relax and assume everything is alright. Stick it out and wait for medical assistance. Only trust the green signal the doctors give you because they know the condition of the patient and whether or not the patient has recovered from the attack.

- Step 5: In the case of open wounds on the chest area or on the neck, you must take care of them immediately. You cannot ignore open wounds in a condition such as this. You can use bandages to cover up the open wounds. In some cases, the wounds start to show air bubbles which usually appear in open wounds. Cover them up with bandages as soon as you can because exposing them and leaving them open is not good.

- Step 6: In the case of a "sucking" chest open wound you must remember the fact that air can get sucked into the cavity and enter the lungs. This type of injury can be one of the reasons why a collapsed lung occurs. The first thing to do in a situation like this would be to bandage or cover the wound using a plastic wrap or a plastic bag. In some cases, people also use gauze pads that are covered in petroleum jelly. The bandage is wrapped around the chest but one part of the bag is not sealed. In this way the air is expelled from the lungs. The covering or the bandage prevents any air from getting into the lungs so that the person does not suffer from a collapsed lung.

When you are tending to a patient who is suffering from Collapsed Lung, be careful not to give him/ her any kind of food or drink. Do not place a pillow or anything at all under the person's head as it can end up blocking the airways. Also, be mindful of not moving the person unless it is absolutely necessary to do so. Do not delay in calling for medical assistance because at any time the person's situation can become worse.

When Do I Need Medical Assistance?

It is often hard to determine when a person with a collapsed lung can be treated at home or when they have to be taken to the hospital for professional medical assistance. Sometimes people just think the symptoms are side effects of the medication and they ignore the signs that tell them they need to rush to the hospital. In order to prevent any dangerous scenarios, here is a guide that helps you determine when you need to rush to the hospital and when you need to call for medical assistance:

- Pain in the chest

- Lightheadedness

- Dizziness

- Excessive drooling

- Blue lips

- Blue fingernails

- Blue fingers

- Hives on the body

- Excessive sweating

- Any nausea or vomiting

- High-pitched sounds whilstbreathing

- Wheezing sounds whilst breathing

- Coughing up large amounts of blood

- Irregular or rapid heartbeat

- The inability to speak at all

- Facial Swelling

- Throat Swelling

- Tongue Swelling

- Shortness of breath, especially when it is brought on by coughing

- Fever

- Cough has a barking sound

- Weight loss is noticeable

Can I Take Part in Physical Activities with Collapsed Lungs?

This question is valid from patients who suffer from Collapsed Lung. Since the lungs are very actively involved in all forms and kinds of exercises, the question raised makes a lot of sense and carries a lot of weight. Whenever you are working out, running, jogging or lifting weights, you will often find yourself out of breath. In addition to that, you will also notice that your breathing patterns become different when you work out as opposed to when you are sitting idle or doing normal day to day work. This is because your lungs and your breathing patterns play an important role when you exercise or carry out strenuous activities in other fields.

Physical activities not only include work out sessions, in fact, physical activities can consist of a number of things that can have an effect on the health of our lungs. These physical activities can be:

- Dancing

- Running and jogging

- Coming up and down the stairs

- Playing games

- Jumping

- Rock Climbing

- Working out

- Cycling

- Swimming

These are only a few examples of physical activities that give rise to the question of whether they can be done or not when a person is suffering from Collapsed Lung. However, this question can be best answered by your doctor, as he or she is completely familiar with your case.

Nevertheless, with a more general analysis, we can conclude that it is usually not very safe for people who have a collapsed lung to take part in the activities listed above.

As it has already been mentioned before, a patient who is suffering from Collapsed Lung needs to go on with his or her life. They need to go and do their day to day activities and then come back home and live a normal life, but in some cases it is best to be careful. Doing all of these activities has a very prominent effect on the lungs, which is why it is advised to avoid them.

Do's And Don'ts

Living with Collapsed Lung is not easy. Even if you have gone through some treatment, the fear that your lungs can collapse even while you are asleep is not only unsettling, it puts a huge question mark 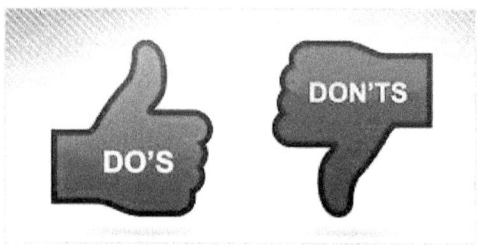 on life. There are hundreds of people all over the world who have fallen victim to Spontaneous Pneumothorax for no fault of their own.

A number of examples and patient experiences given in the book are proof that before a victim walks into an ER, they wait a long time for the symptoms of Collapsed Lung to wear off naturally. Intense coughing, frequent breathlessness and stabbing pains in the chest, back, shoulder and arms are some of the most interfering and crippling signs of Pneumothorax that make it hard for a person to live with partially functioning lungs.

Perhaps, the second most frequently voiced concern among Pneumothorax patients- apart from the reasons for its onset- is the way to take care of it. Many cases of lung collapse are minor and do not need treatment beyond strict observation. In such a situation the patient feels that they are constantly living with Pneumothorax because the chances that it will recur are as high as 25% in most healthy people.

Another instance of living with Collapsed Lung is when Secondary Pneumothorax patients are waiting for treatment. There is a high possibility that because of an underlying lung disease, the most effective Pneumothorax treatment cannot be used for patients with SSP due to a risk of increased complications. Therefore, the waiting period that is characterized with difficulty in breathing and frequent pain, has to be borne with patience and hope.

What should you do to avoid its onset again ? What precautions can you take to make sure living with these lungs does not turn into a condition that is unbearable? There are many Do's and Don'ts that should be kept in mind at all times when living with a collapsed lung and these tips have to be implemented in your daily life for Pneumothorax to become a far off possibility.

Do's:

1. Take plenty of rest if you are living with a collapsed lung. A collapse below 15% is usually treated with observation and rest, therefore, make it a point to put a lot of engagements on hold because your body needs to recuperate and get its energy back before it can fall into the same pattern of daily activities.

2. If you are a SSP patient, get medical help for the underlying lung disease. It is important that this crucial organ of the body is healthy and supplying oxygen to all parts of the body. Pulmonary diseases like cancer weaken the lungs, because of which the development of tears and the rupture of blisters become all the more common. Therefore, if you want the collapse to cease for good, the lungs have to heal completely.

3. If you have had a Pneumothorax surgery, it is imperative that you take care of the wounds. Make sure they are cleaned and dressed every day, or as instructed by the doctor. Moreover, the site of the wound should be kept dry at all times. This ensures the prevention of infections and bacteria.

4. Follow the doctor's advice and directions strictly and make sure you go in for follow ups as soon as they are prescribed by them. Regular observation is one of the most trusted ways to monitor Pneumothorax and to make sure its signs and symptoms do not get out of hand.

5. Get fresh air as much as possible. Unpleasant and harsh environments are not suitable for a patient living with a collapsed lung because they force the lungs to breathe faster and heavily, thus increasing the chances of a collapse. If you are not allowed to exercise a lot, you can enjoy the pleasant weather from a park bench as well.

6. If you have an occupation that puts you in direct danger of suffering from Pneumothorax, you should inform your doctor immediately. For instance, if you are a pilot or a diving

instructor, Lung Collapse can take a totally different meaning and even insist upon a lifestyle or profession switch. Therefore, present all information when you are under diagnosis.

Don'ts:

1. Do not travel via plane immediately after suffering with Pneumothorax or after treatment. Studies suggest that the difference in air pressure is a prominent factor in the occurrence of Lung Collapse. Therefore, pressure changes have to be avoided so that no more air leaks into the chest cavity.

2. Activities like Scuba Diving and Snorkeling are out of the question for a Pneumothorax patient who still needs a lot of care. Both of these activities, in particular, and others like it in general, put the body under stress, urging it to survive on an irregular supply of oxygen. Moreover, longer and deeper breathing can also harm the already weakened walls of the lungs further.

3. Don't smoke at all. Even if you feel the urge to blow a few puffs, you have to restrain yourself because 91% of all Pneumothorax patients have been found to be either active or passive smokers. Smoking after the occurrence of a collapse can raise havoc in the body and disrupt the process of re-inflation of the lungs.

4. Weight lifting is a very strenuous exercise that puts a lot of pressure on the chest cavity, making it hard for the lungs to keep pace. There are numerous instances of Pneumothorax in which the victim felt the first stab of pain in the chest during a heavy weight lifting regime.

5. Do not ignore signs and symptoms. If you are currently living with a partially functioning lung, make sure you keep a watchful eye on how you feel every few hours. An increase in pain or escalation of breathing problems should not be taken lightly under any circumstances.

Tips for Close Friends and Family

Advanced Care Planning

In its advanced stages, Pneumothorax can be crippling. Just like other Chronic Obstructive Lung Diseases, a lung collapse can have a huge impact on the quality of life. While initial stages of Pneumothorax can be treated and cured with outpatient procedures, in patients, who have a history of chronic pulmonary disorders, may find that a lung collapse surgery or chest tube isnot a viable option.

In such a case, the patient may be given relaxants and pain relieving medication, but would not qualify for an intrusive procedure that can cure the collapse for good. Therefore, advanced care planning among family members is a must.

Characterized by wheezing, intense coughing and acute shortness of breath, an advanced case of lung collapse, coupled with other pulmonary diseases, can be extremely crippling for the individual. Daily chores like making meals, doing laundry, cleaning the house or going out to buy supplies can become uphill tasks that the patient cannot manage alone at all.

Chronic diseases, pulmonary in particular, are therefore known to afflict one person but affect the entire family or household. For this reason, the role played by family caregivers is paramount and an indication of the quality of life the patient will now have. Every single member of the household becomes involved when one person goes through an advanced lung collapse condition.

Arranging and planning for care giving at home can be a bit of a hassle at first, after all a lot of preparation has to be done to make sure all the supplies and necessary equipment are present, however, there is no place like home, especially for a patient. Ask a hospitalized person what they want the most and they won't hesitate to express their wish to go home immediately. Therefore, the care given in one's home can make a lot of difference to the extent of the disease and its prevention.

It should be remembered that a chronic lung patient needs ongoing care; a day or two of care planning is not enough because when doctors tell a lung patient to go and live as comfortably as possible, it means there is no other treatment plan available except exceptional care and love. Therefore, when you plan this care regime, make sure you discuss it with the patient and get their approval because their comfort and health are of first priority.

How can caregivers' best care for the patient? How can the patient's quality of life be improved as much as possible? There are many factors and determinants of caregiving that have to be kept in mind when a family or a group of close friends are trying to do as much as possible for a loved one. If you are the head caregiver, there is a lot you need to plan.

The following is a step by step guide to make sure you have everything you need to care for a loved one at home.

- First of all, think about proximity. Do you stay with the patient? If not, being far can be an issue when it comes to regular and proper care. With proximity, you have the added advantage of keeping an eye on every activity and guiding the patient with what to do and what to avoid. Moreover, as mentioned previously, helping with daily chores like cooking, eating, changing clothes and moving around can only be done when you live with or live very close to the patient.

  If you do not, however, you can hire a full time nurse to help?

- Second, you need a supply of medicines. Pulmonary disease patients are on strict doses of medication because the lungs and their capacity have to be maintained for adequate breathing. When you decide to take care of your patient, contact the doctor who has made the diagnosis to get a prescription of all the medications you will need to stock up at home. Make sure they are located close to where the patient spends most of their time and the doses are clearly marked on them.

- Now you need some equipment. Lung disease patients are often tied to an oxygen supply that aids their breathing and inflates the lungs to their maximum potential. Even though the supply doesn't have to be constantly attached, taking external oxygen

74

is encouraged by doctors so that the body is not put under a lot of breathing stress. Hence, make sure you have an oxygen supply on standby and you are aware of how to use the equipment, if need be.

- Daily exercises. Not all patients are required to rest all the time. You will have to inquire how your patient needs to spend their day. Ask the doctor if any exercises are allowed. If they are, make sure you learn which ones, because you will have to help the patient perform the steps exactly as they should be. Set aside a time and duration for exercise or walking so that they can be done in a regular pattern.

- A huge portion of home care is about making the patient comfortable and loved. Spend time with the individual, talk about their favorite topics, their likes and dislikes and what they find the most soothing when it comes to Pneumothorax treatment. If you live far, make sure you take out some time during the day to visit and interact with your loved one on a daily basis. Being lonely and alienated is the worst feeling that can make a sick person progress in the illness at a much accelerated rate.

The steps outlined above are only the very basic ones that you need to prepare for, physically and mentally. After this planning phase, the real work begins. Once you have everything in place, you will now do Disease Management and Intervention- which are parts of advanced care giving because they involve in-home steps to minimize breathing discomfort.

Being the primary caregiver, always make sure that you are ready to take any steps toward enhancing the comfort of the patient so that their life can be improved in any way possible.

Disease Management and Intervention

As a caregiver, you have to be well versed with the condition that plagues the patient under your care. Despite being a family member, a friend or a relative, if you have taken the responsibility to provide immediate and direct care for an individual with Collapsed Lung, Disease Management comes under your job description.

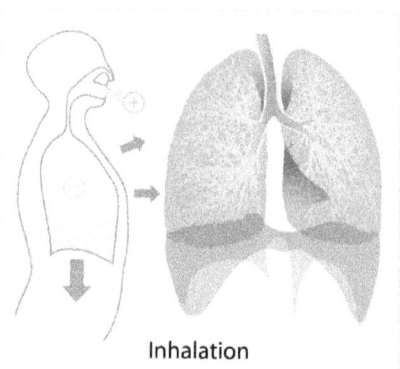

Inhalation

What is Disease Management and Intervention? To understand this concept, you first have to tell yourself that taking care of a pulmonary patient is not a small thing, nor is it based on trial and errors. It is a systematic process that has to be repeated day after day, with progress being recorded at regular intervals. Hence, Disease Management and Intervention *"is a system that aims to take care of and manage chronic ailments of high-risk and high-cost patients."*

For the implementation of this system, the planning process discussed above has to be in place, together with a serious and unwavering attitude for the well-being of the patient. For you to be able to perform Disease Management for a lung collapse patient, you have to be vigilant, alert and highly committed to this altruistic job.

Since DM is a systematic process, what are the steps that make it up? How can you manage these steps and how can you make sure they lead to betterment and progress for your loved one? Let's break down the details of Disease Management for Pulmonary Ailments so that you can implement them for your patient.

We suggest that you put these steps in writing so that if you are unavailable, the paramedics or any other caregiver can take your place in an emergency. Lastly, discuss all these steps with your loved one. Make sure the patient is aware of the Disease Management steps and you have their full consent. By keeping the patient on board, you will ensure that all the emergency steps are in their mind as well. This will help them to stay calm by eliminating uncertainty.

Step 1: Keep a Log

Now that you are fully aware of your patient's ailment and have the necessary equipment and medication needed, the first step is to draft a daily log in which progress will be recorded. This log will be a daily journal in which you write down all information related to the patient. To maintain it, you have to ensure that regular entries are made and all reported signs and symptoms are recorded.

This way, when the doctor calls the patient for a follow up, you will be able to give an accurate account of how well they are doing and the problems encountered since they were diagnosed. This daily log should contain information such as:

- Names of all medications, their doses, times and side effects.

- Symptoms experienced before, after- or in many cases without any treatment as well. Note down whether the patient feels pain at certain times or while doing certain activities etc.

- The diet being followed. How do they feel with the diet?

- Any exercise done and at what times.

- Pattern of breathing. Is it hard to breathe normally? Does it hurt? Instances of breathlessness should also be recorded.

Step 2: When to Seek Medical Help

A Pneumothorax can occur spontaneously at any time, during the day or night. Symptoms can get worse and new signs of a collapse can appear out of nowhere. Hence, knowing when to call the doctor and get help is important for a caregiver.

The onset of a collapse cripples the patient with pain and intense coughing, making it impossible for them to take any steps on their own. Therefore, it will be your responsibility to ring up a doctor, nurse or the ER and ask for help. If the following symptoms are experienced, you should seek help.

- Swelling in hands, feet and ankles.

- Increased difficulty in breathing, followed by a fit of painful dry cough.

- Spitting of mucus that has blood. It may also have an odor and a greenish color.

- Unbearable chest pain.

- Intense fatigue and muscle cramps.

- Breathlessness that doesn't let the patient fall asleep.

- Distress symptoms that are out of the ordinary and are not seen on a daily basis.

Step 3: Do Not Panic

If your loved one is in distress for the first time since surgery or the last collapse, for instance, there is a high chance that you will go into panic mode. Losing your wits will make the situation an even bigger emergency. If you detect these warning signs in the patient, you should calm yourself down and take a few minutes to get ready to act.

Moreover, you can also call a friend or another family member for additional help and emotional support. If you have a 24 hour nurse hired for the patient, you can wake him/her up and discuss the situation as well. If you stay calm and hopeful, you can tell your loved one to do the same as well.

Step 4: Who to Call?

Being the primary caregiver, you should know who to contact in the time of need. Before you sign up for the job, you should ideally accompany the patient on one of their trips to the doctor they see so that you can take their contact details for emergency situations.

In the same journal that you use to record progress, clearly note down the contact information, extensions and pager details of the doctors you are suppose to stay in touch with. You can also put this information on the fridge or a notice board in the kitchen where everyone can find it easily.

In short, no time should be wasted looking for the doctor's business card because this crucial piece of information should be readily available.

Step 5: Emergency Steps

When you call the doctor, nurse or the ER, you will be told what to do. Sometimes, if the onset of these symptoms is predicted by the doctors, you will not be told to bring the patient in for a checkup. Instead, the doctor may give you instructions and an altered treatment plan so that you can help your loved one in this time.

Before doing so, they will ask you a bit about the situation at hand and how the patient has been progressing in the last few weeks. At this time, keep your daily log with you so you can update the doctor regarding the patient's condition and everything they have felt in the days leading up to the emergency.

After hearing this information, the doctor can give either one or all of the following instructions:

- Change of medication. Write down the new medicines and corresponding doses that the doctor prescribes.

- Specific exercises. You may be told that to treat the patient requires a particular way to relieve some pain and discomfort.

- Specific instructions. The doctor may tell you to monitor the patient for a duration of time and if the symptoms persist, they should be taken to the ER. Make sure you take note of all these instructions so you can provide the best emergency care.

Step 6: Accompany the Patient to the Hospital

If the doctor tells you to bring the patient to the hospital, make sure you accompany them. Being the primary caregiver, your information and observation of the patient will be extremely valuable to the ER doctors who will do the preliminary assessments and tests.

Some of the most important details you will be asked are: when the symptoms occurred, how long has the patient been in this condition, was it sudden or not, changes in the color of their mucus if any, what was their pattern of breathing and intensity of chest pains in the hours leading up to the emergency?

Maximizing Family Care

Giving care and love to a Pneumothorax patient at home requires a lot of physical and emotional effort. Seeing a loved one go through so much pain, exertion and discomfort is not only hard, it can weaken the strongest of people. However, in cases where little can be done by hospitalizing the patient, home care is the best remedy to help the patient progress towards betterment.

However, none of this is to say that the primary caregiver is not a human. Being at the beck and call of a patient can take a toll on you very easily. If it isn't the physical work, it will be the emotional effort of keeping high spirits and hope in front of them. If you are looking after a minor to mild case of Pneumothorax, in high probability, the patient's condition will improve within 15 days and your efforts will pay off.

However, if the case is one of SSP or a major lung collapse, the symptoms may worsen day by day. In this situation, your job as a caregiver may be permanent or consume a lot of your time on a daily basis – meaning giving you very few opportunities to be on your own and tend to your own life. It is common sense that a patient can be well taken care of only when the caregiver is in top shape, physically and mentally.

Therefore, while you take care of your sick loved one, you have to look after yourself too to maximize the care you provide.

Tips for Caregivers

- Uncertainty can be daunting. Make sure you are well aware of your responsibilities. Study the signs and symptoms and follow all of the instructions given by the doctors or nurses to make sure you haven't left out any important information.

- Do some research. Being at the top of your game whilst giving care is the best way to make sure you are prepared for emergencies and unprecedented events. Research on the onset of lung collapse, what to do when it does and how to deal with it before help arrives.

- Contact the hospital to inquire about health care services that can aid you in taking care of the patient. Joining support groups for patients with similar problems can be a great way to buck up and look forward to a hopeful future. It can also help you understand the problems facing your loved one better and how to deal with them.

- Try to not be the only one taking care of the patient. Call on friends, other family members and neighbors who are willing to pitch in some effort. Take turns to run errands and spend time with the patient so that none of the caregivers tire out.

- Read up on patient experiences and personal stories to see how others have 'been there, done that.' This can give caregivers a true insight into how to make a difference in someone else's life.

- Make sure you take adequate rest and breaks from time to time so that your resolve doesn't suffer. If you have an event to attend, hire a sitter or ask another family member to volunteer and help, while you take some time out. Cutting away from social life can be a big damper on your spirits.

- If you prefer to do the patient's work all by yourself, hire help for other chores like cooking, cleaning or babysitting; any help in this regard will take some burden off you so that you can devote time and effort to yourself as well without getting tired of working doubly hard.

- Bring new changes to your lifestyle. To distract yourself while your loved one is asleep or resting, you can meditate. Meditation has been proven as a relaxing exercise that helps the mind, body and heart in recuperating and re-energizing.

- If, despite all your efforts and dedication, the patient is not being taken care of well enough, make an informed decision. Perhaps a nursing home or assisted living facility is the best option for those who are extremely old, need undivided attention or have too many problems that cannot be handled at home without proper training. Even though such a decision is hard to make, it may be in the best interest of your loved one.

Online Resources for Patients

As Pneumothorax has become a more common condition over the years, it has received a lot of attention from medical professionals and those conducting research and studies in medicine. As the results poured in, they were compiled into useful and relevant information for use by patients and experts alike.

Today, the internet is a great resource for acquiring information about Collapsed Lung – a condition that was otherwise hardly ever heard of. From the causes, signs and symptoms to the most important precautions and prevention tips, every little detail is available on the World Wide Web.

Like any other practice, medical techniques and procedures differ from region to region. While there are standards to go by when assessing the extent of Pneumothorax or the treatment methods for patients, there is always a difference of opinion in every diagnosis and its analysis.

Moreover, the resources cited also have to take into consideration the local clinics, hospitals and other caregiving facilities, so that patients can make use of the information. Therefore, information regarding Pneumothorax should be taken from websites that are specific to the region you belong to.

As a broad classification, the following are online resources for all kinds of information on Collapsed Lung from three main regions, namely Europe, the United States and the United Kingdom.

Resources for the UK

- Patient.co.uk

  http://www.patient.co.uk/doctor/pneumothorax-pro

- British Lung Foundation

  http://www.blf.org.uk/Conditions/Detail/Pneumothorax

- Royal Berkshire

  http://www.royalberkshire.nhs.uk/patient-information-leaflets/pneumothorax-august-2013.htm

- Bleb Info

  http://www.blebinfo.co.uk/phpBB2/portal.php

Resources for the US

- NY Times Health Guide

  http://www.nytimes.com/health/guides/disease/pneumothorax/overview.html

- Mayo Clinic

  http://www.mayoclinic.org/diseases-conditions/pneumothorax/basics/definition/con-20030025

- Medicine Net

  http://www.medicinenet.com/pneumothorax/article.htm

- Up To Date

  http://www.uptodate.com/contents/primary-spontaneous-pneumothorax-in-adults

- Mount Sinai Medical Center

  http://sinaiem.us/tutorials/pneumothorax

Resources for Europe

- Europe Pub Med Central

  http://europepmc.org/articles/PMC3982243

- European Society of Thoracic Surgeons

  http://www.ests.org/guidelines_and_evidence/guideline_databa
  se.aspx

While information on these sites is accurate, always make it a point to run it by your general physician. Since it is necessary to be sure that what you have read applies to your Pneumothorax case, it is important to keep your doctor on board before you take any step.

Moreover, these resources also contain helpful guides that assist you in determining whether your condition is similar to Pneumothorax or not. Knowing about this condition as much as possible is the best way to detect early signs and catch it in the initial stages before it becomeshighly painful.

Curing Pneumothorax: How Long Does It Take

After Surgery Effects

Surgery for Pneumothorax, being the most invasive treatment for Pneumothorax, results in many post-operative effects that have to be dealt with patiently. A lot of care is needed after Pleurisies is performed on a Collapsed Lung patient because it takes quite some time for the wounds to heal and for the body to adjust to the new internal changes.

Generally, the extent of post-operative effects and care needed are directly related to the type of surgery performed and the severity of the collapse. For instance, if the surgery can be completed with a sprinkling of a talc-like irritant, the body will adapt to it sooner than it will adapt to the changes made if the entire pleural space is obliterated.

Therefore, while post-surgical effects vary from case to case, it is safe to assume that every Pneumothorax related surgery will have a series of aftercare situations that will require a lot of patience and sensitivity on the part of caregivers. According to medical experts, complications and negative effects of the surgery are most likely to show up from Day 1 to Day 3 after the surgery.

During this time the patient is kept under strict observation, with regular monitoring of the lungs and their adaptability to the new internal conditions. Some very common complications that can arise post surgery include the following. It helps to remember that most of these are witnessed in cases where the Pneumothorax is very severe.

1. Post Operative Fever – Fever is a direct effect of any kind of surgery. With Pneumothorax, the chances of getting a fever are high because the surgery involves stabilizing the pressure of air inside the body. Until Day 2, the patient may experience mild fever which is quite normal. However, if the fever becomes persistent beyond Day 4, the doctor may investigate the reason for this complication. Fever resulting from surgery is usually a signal that the body is reacting to the internal changes. It is the

sum total of all side effects and reactions in the postoperative period.

2. Hemorrhage – Hemorrhage is another likely result of surgery if the patient has bled a lot before, during or after it. Many a times, a hemorrhage is caused by internal bleeding of a suture if the tear on the lung has not been repaired properly or there has been further rupture of blisters.

    Compared to fever, hemorrhages have to be taken care of immediately, because they can create havoc in the patient's body. Blood clots can increase blood pressure in the arteries and prevent the supply of oxygen and blood to various body parts. Postoperative hemorrhage in Pneumothorax patients can be a result of damaged blood vessels around the site of incision.

    To make sure minor clots are kept in check, doctors often advise regular blood tests, platelet counts and clotting screens to make sure that the hemorrhage dissolves on its own. However, if it does not, another surgery may be needed. Such a surgery is exploratory in nature, to find the source of hemorrhage and fix it.

3. Infection – Developing an infection is another common post-surgery effect. Since a surgery involves the use of metallic knives and tongs on the inner flesh of the body, the chances of getting an infection are very high. In fact, the extensive care given to Pneumothorax patients after surgery is primarily to keep a check on infection development. The most common type of infection in this regard is a wound infection, which is characterized by redness, superficial pain and discharge from the wound on the chest.

    Therefore, keeping the wound clean and changing bandages at regular intervals are two of the prescribed prevention tips to reduce the chances of post-surgery infections.

4. Unstable Wound Healing – Very slow and irregular wound healing may also occur after the surgery. This isn't to say that wounds post Pneumothorax surgery don't heal properly. Sometimes the incision site heals within a day or two, however,

in some cases, it takes a while before the wounds are stabilized. Some common reasons for this are:

- Tension in the sutures

- Poor blood supply

- Vitamin deficiency

- Infections

5. Surgical Injury – While performing surgery, needles and scalpels can sometimes cause more harm than good. This is why only the most professional surgeons should be allowed to perform invasive surgeries like the one for Pneumothorax. Apart from this, the instances of unavoidable tissue damage are also very frequent. For instance, if the collapsed lung is to be stitched to the chest wall, some tissues of the wall and the organ are bound to get scarred.

6. Respiratory Complications – After a surgery for Collapsed Lungs, it can take some time for the lungs to start functioning normally. Experiencing minor discomfort and irritation while breathing is a common post-surgery effect, which eases in a few days. In case the patient feels uneasy even afterwards, the complication can be discussed amongst a panel of doctors.

Bowel Related Problems – While the body adjusts to the new conditions, the bowel may become irritated. One particular post surgery effect that is high on a doctor's list is the passage of waste from the body. Even if the bowel system is disrupted, the doctor will make sure your fiber intake is high and that urine is

7. passing out regularly. If this is not the case, the chances of infection are very high.

8. Drug Reaction– Allergies and instant reactions to medication are constantly monitored before and after surgery. However, sometimes drug reactions occur despite the level of care a patient is given. Because the body goes through tremendous stress and pressure during surgery, it can react badly to drugs as a way of showing its discomfort.

Things to Remember

Once a few days have passed since the Pneumothorax treatment was performed on you, the doctors can agree to let you go home. At this point, you will not be fully recovered. Therefore, though you will be allowed to leave the hospital, special care instructions will be given to make sure that post-surgery effects do not cause Pneumothorax to recur.

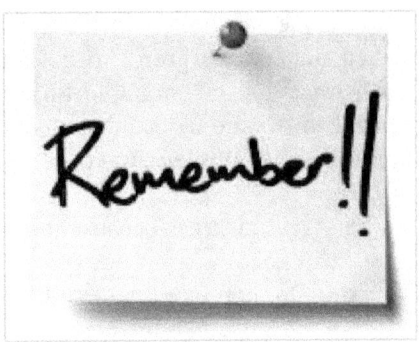

Many patients with a collapsed lung who have been treated via a chest tube are sent home after a day or two, with the tube still intact. In this case, the chest tube has to be taken care of at home by your family or other caregivers who will be present 24/7 to look after you. Walking, bending, turning and settling into a daily routine is particularly hard with a chest tube and a bottle in tow. Hence, you have to remember to be extra cautious so that the equipment attached to your body is not disturbed in any way.

A few things to remember in this case are:

- Always carry the attached bottle and chest tube with you when you get up and walk.

- Make sure no pressure is applied to the tube, otherwise its position will be altered.

- Since the tube is inserted in your side, there is an incision under the armpit that has to be taken care of. Ensure that the wound is dry and clean at all times. Developing an infection at the site of the incision is very easy if the wound is left wet or if the dressing is not changed regularly.

- Moreover, the doctor will give instructions regarding the monitoring of the tube as well. If the tube oozes blood or any type of liquid, it should be reported immediately because the only purpose of the chest tube is to suck out excess air.

In cases where the patient has been treated surgically, the body will be going through a complete revamping of its system, as it tries to cope with the added stress and pressure of surgery. Many patients prefer to stay in the hospital until the bandage is off and the tubes, if any, are taken out; others prefer to go home and be taken care of personally. Either way, it takes ample time for the body to heal completely and during this time a lot of precautions and care instructions have to be kept in mind. While you recover, make sure to remember the following:

- Avoid stress because it accelerates breathing and pulse.

- Do not exert yourself physically. Avoid strenuous exercises because they increase the tension in the chest muscles that need time to heal completely.

- Since your body has gone through a lot, it will feel exhausted and tired after the surgery. You will experience pain in the shoulders, neck and back. This is normal; however, this requires you to take special care so that the pain reduces instead of becoming chronic.

- Avoid air travel for some time because the pressure in the chest cavity needs to remain stable for the lungs to recover.

- Avoid talking or laughing loudly.

- Smoking is now strictly prohibited for you. Exposing the lungs to tobacco will worsen the Pneumothorax and increase its chances of recurring.

- If you have been a victim of SSP, continue taking medication for the lung disease you are suffering from. Consult your doctor for more guidelines.

- Try to stay away from harsh environmental conditions that make it difficult for you to breathe.

- Take ample rest and eat healthy so that the body can recuperate as quickly as possible.

How Long Does It Take?

Recovery from a collapsed lung takes some time. While some people are up and about in record time, others find it hard to cope post-surgery. When a patient is informed that they are suffering from Collapsed Lung, one of the first questions that come to mind is how long will it take for the entire procedure to be performed.

The time taken for a collapsed lung to be treated and for the patient to recover fully depends on various factors. These include the following:

- The type of Pneumothorax: A PSP is known to be milder compared to an SSP attack. Since the patient's condition is already complicated in the latter, it can take more time for them to recover and carry on with everyday activities. On the other hand, people who suffer from Primary Spontaneous Pneumothorax recover faster because they are otherwise healthy.

- Severity of Pneumothorax: If a very mild collapse occurs, it takes less time to heal compared to one that affects more than 50% of the lungs. Hence, the severity of the condition is a big indicator of how long it will take for the patient to get back to normal.

- Procedure performed: The time taken for recovery is directly proportional to the treatment option chosen by the medical expert. Aspiration, for instance, is often performed as an outpatient procedure that can be completed in two to three hours. Once it is completed and the vitals stabilize, patients are allowed to leave with medications and instructions on what to do next. However, if the treatment involves surgery, the time to heal increases significantly because the wounds have to heal before the patient is allowed to carry on with daily activities.

- Lifestyle choices: The lifestyle choices an individual makes also determines how quickly they are able to get back on their feet. For instance, if a smoker who has gone through a chest tube procedure for a collapsed lung doesn't intend to quit, their recovery can be a long and painful process. Similarly, those patients who gradually build up their stamina for healthy exercise after the collapse is treated, are likely to have a fit and healthy body.

Unless major complications arise, a Pneumothorax patient recovers in about 15-20 days on average if the collapse is not very significant in nature. During this period, caregivers are given strict instructions to exercise caution regarding the wounds, incisions, breathing and overall health of the recovering individual.

The factors listed above play a major role in determining the recovery time. If all seems to be in place 2 to 3 days after hospitalization and surgery, doctors become fairly confident in letting the patient recover at a gradual pace in the comfort of their own home and in familiar surroundings.

Patient Experiences

Going through an instance of Collapsed Lung is scary and overwhelming. Seeing a loved one experience the pain and discomfort is equally bad. Being the spontaneous condition that it is, Pneumothorax is often unavoidable and, in many cases, unforeseeable as well. No matter how healthy you might be, it can take as much as a blister rupture, the size of a pea, for a collapse to occur and put your body in stress.

Sometimes doctors fail to pinpoint exactly what spurs this condition and the circumstances under which it subsides. The fact that in many cases the lungs manage to inflate on their own when the air that has leaked into the system escapes, is another mystery of Pneumothorax that makes this condition very hard to put into a strict pattern.

With many facets of Collapsed Lung left up to fate – or the medicine gods – a high level of uncertainty often surrounds this condition. In this situation, a lot of comfort and valuable advice can be drawn from the experiences of those who have already gone though a similar condition. For the mother of a 15 year old boy who may be at risk of Pneumothorax, the valuable words of another woman who has just gone through the same episode with her child can help her feel in control of the situation.

No doubt, every Pneumothorax case varies from person to person; however, drawing similarities from the experiences of others can often help in mentally preparing you for the onset of the condition. Moreover, for many people the advice that comes from someone who has experienced a collapsed lung before is more highly regarded than that of a doctor. These people feel that doctors either do not clarify the situation enough, are sometimes too vague in their answers or worse, are out to scare and overwhelm those inquiring about ailments.

Five Pneumothorax Patients, Five Different Stories

If you are a reader who wants to know about Pneumothorax from those who have had firsthand experience with the condition, reading patient stories should be your next step. However, before we move on to patient experiences, a disclaimer is called for. While these experiences provide valuable insight, always remember that no two cases are the same and hence, the exact treatments and diagnosis can never be standardized across the board.

That said, let's now take a look at how people from various walks of life went through and managed Pneumothorax.

1. Patient Profile- Ramosm: Male, Age 25-34

For Ramosm, Pneumothorax took over while he was exercising in the gym. After lifting a particularly heavy weight, Ramosm felt strained and out of breath. The sudden pain on the right side of his chest seemed out of the ordinary. However, thinking that the pain was just a muscle pull, he spent some time stretching to alleviate it.

Still suffering from breathlessness, Ramosm's colleague pointed out that he looked extremely pale (a very prominent sign of a collapsed lung). It wasn't long before the victim was taken to the closest ER via an ambulance. After a series of X-Rays and preliminary tests, Ramosm was told that his entire right lung had collapsed and too much air in the chest cavity was preventing normal breathing.

To relieve the pain instantly, Ramosm was taken to surgery immediately after the diagnosis. The procedure performed was a combination of Pleurodesis and Bleb Resection to prevent further leakage of air. After being observed for one week, he was informed that the test results were anything but satisfactory. A lot more air had leaked into the chest cavity, and since it was hard to determine why, Ramosm had to be taken for surgery once again.

After a long period of 3 weeks, he was finally discharged after the results came out satisfactory. Ramosm's experience is one that highlights a severe case of lung collapse. Having the entire right side collapse and going through surgery twice, made the Primary Spontaneous Pneumothorax very dangerous and painful.

2. Patient Profile- Evi: Female, Age 30-32

Evi woke up one day from a deep sleep – tired and breathless. Being a healthy mother of three, Evi had no bad habits like smoking or doing drugs. Her health had always been perfect before and after she gave birth to her youngest son. Pneumothorax disrupted Evi's life when the breathlessness continued to plague her for one whole week, after which it turned into a severe, chest gripping dry cough.

Throughout the week that Evi thought these symptoms were only a result of everyday exertion and tiredness, she went through her daily chores; attended gym class, went bowling with her friends and tended to her toddler. However, when the coughing came even in the way of casual small talk, her husband convinced her to see a physician.

For Evi, the diagnosis results were 'the biggest shock of her life.' When the doctor told her she was going through a condition called Pneumothorax – meaning, collapse of the lung – she couldn't believe it. What shocked her to the core was the fact that she had never indulged in any bad habits and was never ill in any way.

Nonetheless, the immediate procedure she went through was chest tube insertion, after which she was transported to the hospital to be admitted. Over a period of 4 days, the air leakage was controlled and when it reduced to 10%, Evi was discharged and allowed to leave with strict instructions to contact immediately if signs and symptoms reappeared.

3. Patient Profile- Eddy: Male, Age 25-34

Eddy's love for basketball landed him in the hospital with a collapsed lung. While on the field, Eddy started feeling pain on the left side of his chest, coupled with intense breathlessness. Unable to continue playing, he was transported to the ER where CT Scans and X-Rays indicated a mild Pneumothorax.

Thankfully, he didn't require surgery or drainage and with the help of calming and relaxing pills, the air rim in the chest reduced from 30% to only 5%. After 5 days he was allowed to go home, however, little did he know that the same collapse would recur and magnify in the next 5 months. The next attack was worse than the previous one, hence, surgery was decided upon.

Even though the Pneumothorax has not recurred, Eddy still feels mild pain on the left side of his chest from time to time, especially during the Winter.

4. Patient Profile- Der: Female, Age 35-44

Der suffered from Pneumothorax as an aftereffect of a double Mastectomy. Being operated upon, she was admitted to the hospital, but at this point, none of it was related to Collapsed Lung. It was after she was discharged that Der felt she became breathless way too often and her right shoulder blade ached badly.

Waiting it out, she let the pain come and go for about a month, after which she went in again for a follow-up for the Mastectomy. It was during this check up that X-rays revealed she was suffering from a collapsed right lung. A chest tube was attached and she was allowed to go home. However, just after two days, the doctors decided that the drainage was not working well enough.

Der went through surgery for Pneumothorax and was admitted to the hospital once again with a number of tubes running from her chest and stomach. Once the painful recovery period ended, Der felt more like her own self – healthy and active.

5. Patient Profile- Jeff: Male, Age 20-25

The type of Pneumothorax that Jeff experienced is classified as a Traumatic Lung Collapse. After falling from the stairs, he fractured 3 ribs that caused his right lung to collapse. Rushed to emergency, at this point the collapse was close to 20%; however, by the time he was tended to it had increased to 75%.

Jeff was unable to breathe, talk or lie still. A chest tube was inserted to release the pressure of air that had built up in his chest. Once he was allowed to go home, Jeff continued with his every day evening walk. However, instead of making him feel better, it worsened the condition of the incision under his armpit when the tube rubbed against the sensitive inner chest wall.

Since then, he has learnt that being as still as possible and getting ample rest with a chest tube is the best way to make sure it is working properly. Once the tube was taken out, Jeff started to feel much better. Soon he was able to fall back into his everyday routine with work, family and a busy lifestyle.

Jeff's experience with Pneumothorax, though traumatic in other ways, was not as severe as the others we have presented. Moreover, his body was able to cope with the stress and his lungs didn't collapse again after the procedure was completed.

Quality Of Life after Surgery

A long and detailed discussion about the postoperative care instructions and patients' personal experiences with Pneumothorax will now be followed by the concerns one might have about the effect of the treatment options on a patient's life. Does Pneumothorax and its remedies affect, enhance 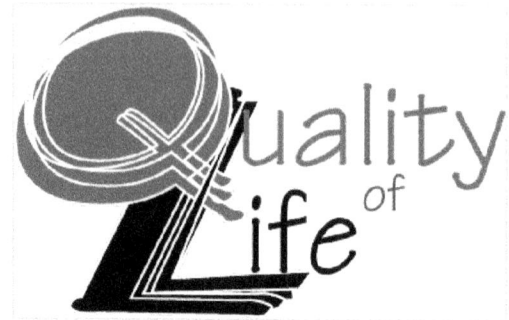 or reduce the quality of life in any way? How can this effect be reversed, if possible, or minimized so that the individual can enjoy life as it was before the condition occurred?

These are some of the most important questions related to the impact of Pneumothorax on the quality of life of a patient. Since this is a topic of concern for medical professionals and caregivers, extensive study, research and surveys have been conducted to draw conclusions. One such study will be discussed in this topic because it gives clear evidence of what patients felt post-surgery and how they planned to live life ahead.

An assessment of the quality of life (QoL) not only gives food for thought for Pulmonologists, it also makes room for improvement in the treatments used for the condition. For these reasons, the QoL assessment has become one of the most important barometers of success in the treatment of Pneumothorax.

According to the Oxford Journal, an extensive QoL study used a questionnaire for the assessment, and was conducted on a total of 20 patients, approved for International Cancer Studies. This questionnaire has been drafted by the European Organization for Research and Treatment of Cancer and contains 30 questions – all of which are structured differently. While it has been used for QoL assessments for various diseases, being a lung disorder, Pneumothorax could also benefit from the survey.

To make the study comprehensive and complete, the questionnaire was mailed to the patients before surgery/treatment and four times after treatment during the 1st, 3rd, 6th and 12th month of surgery. The results of the questionnaire revealed that most patients expressed a very poor QoL before surgery because of intense coughing, breathlessness and acute pain that robbed them of the ability to perform day to day activities.

The results of the research showed that a majority of the patients took the surgery quite well. Their tolerance level for the pain and discomfort was high and the QoL generally increased over the postoperative 12 months. The same study also broke down the analysis by questioning patients on the type of treatment option performed on them. VAT (Video-assisted Thoracoscopic Pleurectomy), a state-of-the-art procedure, yielded the best results because it was minimally invasive and the patients were able to get on their feet in a shorter period of time.

However, on the other hand, another study confirmed that almost 32% of the 60 patients questioned who had undergone surgery for Pneumothorax, complained of postoperative pain even after months had gone by. Therefore, even though the results of different studies vary, a general trend and pattern of the QoL of Pneumothorax patients suggest that the more technologically advanced a surgical procedure is, the better the QoL that patients enjoyed post-surgery.

Current Developments Regarding Pneumothorax

A Look into Past and Present Research

Being a disease that affects one of the most important organs of the body, Pneumothorax and its treatments have attracted a lot of attention in medical circles. Even though a lot is still vague and uncertain about this condition, science has evolved enough to give answers and explanations regarding the majority of lung collapse cases that are reported.

Just like any other disease, Pneumothorax has been researched upon in great detail – more so because of its spontaneous nature. Pulmonologists and general surgeons alike have spent countless hours digging out facts and figures and conducting experiments to establish some reason as to why it occurs and how it can be cured.

Every development regarding this ailment that we hear about today is a result of years of research and hard work put in by medical experts to help doctors diagnose and treat lung collapses better. However, this isn't to say that all conclusions drawn from these studies have value today, because with time, many have been revised, refuted or replaced with even better ones.

Therefore, it wouldn't be wrong to say that Pneumothorax – as a medical condition – has gone through a development curve. Let's take a look at some past and present research and the general progression that has been witnessed in this area of Pulmonology over the years.

I. Atmospheric Variation And Pneumothorax – A Groundbreaking Causal Relationship

In 1988, when very little was known about the collapsed state of the lungs, groundbreaking research was carried out by a group of researchers, who experimented the causal relationship between atmospheric pressure and Pneumothorax. The study was initiated with the hypothesis that Spontaneous Pneumothorax was a result of the rupture of blebs in the chest cavity.

Moreover, it was established that their rupture was caused by the changes in atmospheric pressure, which was symbolized as (ΔAP). Therefore, to confirm this relationship, the study took into account two variables, Air Pressure (ΔAP) and the onset of SP. Data for (ΔAP) was collected by using a 36 year record of atmospheric pressure and its changes, while for SP, the admissions data of 192 SP patients in the last 5 years at a nearby hospital were studied.

Limits to the Research

To narrow the scope of the research as much as possible, which would in turn increase the chances of getting targeted results, a few limits were set in place. These included:

- Changes in the atmospheric pressure for only four days prior to when the collapses were observed.

- Limits for (ΔAP) were defined such that a fall below the 5th percentile and a rise above the 95th percentile was regarded abnormal. This meant that if SP occurred when the pressure dropped below this limit or rose above this limit, the hypothesis would be confirmed.

- Traumatic Pneumothorax was excluded.

The Results

The results of the research can be summarized as follows:

- A majority of 72% of Collapsed Lung cases were subject to abnormal air pressures on at least one of the 4 days. Symptoms and distress signs began to show after this exposure.

- Those who were exposed to more than 4 abnormal air pressure instances, experienced Pneumothorax symptoms more frequently.

Conclusion

The study provided evidence regarding the occurrence of Pneumothorax in relation to changes in air pressure. However, this relationship could not be established with a lot of certainty. While a correlation did exist, it only proved that (ΔAP) was one of the factors that have the power to spur a collapsed lung. The researchers concluded that there were many other factors that governed this condition; however, they were able to say, with certainty, that the rupture of blebs was a definite factor in this equation.

This study, though short on conclusiveness, became food for thought for many others that came after it. It laid the foundation of the entire thought process that links a collapsed lung to the air pressures in the Pleural space and within other organs of the body.

II. Detecting Occult Pneumothorax With Revolutionary CT Scans

This study, conducted in 2007, explains the instance of Occult Pneumothorax and the evolutionary way to detect it. Until a few years ago, the most widely used diagnostic tool to detect a collapsed lung was X-Ray. Easy and quick to perform, X-Rays exposed the inner conditions of the body for doctors who then examined these to detect the source of air leakage and the condition of the lungs in the chest cavity.

However, as many Collapsed Lung cases recurred, the efficacy of this diagnostic tool was put under interrogation. Medical experts and observers decided that X-Rays alone were unable to give a complete and comprehensive analysis of the chest cavity, leading to inconclusive Pneumothorax diagnoses that were sometimes more harmful than no detection at all.

Occult Pneumothorax is a collapse that cannot be detected by an X-Ray. Therefore, the use of CT Scans was made compulsory so that even the smallest tear on the lung walls became visible.

Research Specifics

- The presence of Occult Pneumothorax was studied in Trauma patients only.

- 21,193 trauma patients were observed.

- Patients with or without chest tubes were included in the study.

The Results

To confirm the presence of Occult Pneumothorax, doctors studied X-Ray films of the patients who were part of the study. A Scoring System was then drafted which quantified the size of the Occult Pneumothorax. While the technicalities of the study are out of the scope of this literature, it suffices to understand that X-Rays that matched a certain score were classified as instances of Occult Pneumothorax.

The distance of the largest air pocket measured from the chest wall was the base measurement used for the Scoring System. From the 21,193 patients observed, 1295 had developed Pneumothorax and out of these, 379 were confirmed for Occult collapse. 95.7% of Occult Pneumothorax occurred after trauma and the overall instance of this condition was 1.8%.

Conclusion

Depending on the size of the Occult Pneumothorax, treatment options were discussed for patients. This study uncovered an important finding that the chances of going through a collapse that cannot be diagnosed via an X-Ray are quite high. Therefore, this tool should only be used in conjunction with other more advanced procedures like CT Scans.

III.   Does Pneumothorax Lead To Pulmonary Oedema?

The scope of this study, conducted in 2014, is quite wide because it explores the nature of Pneumothorax as a condition that can have lasting effects. It answers a very pertinent question regarding the results of Pneumothorax, i.e. its duration is a factor determining the damage caused to lungs.

The research aimed to establish a link between Pneumothorax treatment (its specifics) and lung damage. Specifically, two factors in Lung Collapse were studied; one, whether the duration of the collapse affects the lung adversely and two, whether the drainage of air from the chest cavity causes Oedema.

Research Specifics

- The two variations of duration were 30 minutes and 5 minutes, while those for Drainage were Drained (D) or Not Drained (ND).

- The study was conducted on rats because the deliberate delay in air drainage can be risky for humans.

The Results and Conclusion

The Rats were first given anesthesia and then an air rim was injected in their chest cavity using syringes. The results concluded that rats in the D group differed in the extent of lung damage, which was directly proportional to the delay experienced in air drainage. Those that were tested for 30 minutes showed less Oedema and hyperinflation, suggesting that the quicker a Pneumothorax is treated, the better the chances that a lung can be re-inflated with minimal damage.

Conclusion

If you had previously never heard of a condition called Pneumothorax, you will now be well versed with it. There is a lot of know about Lung Collapse because this condition, and its treatments, have evolved over the years greatly. The way Pneumothorax was looked upon previously has changed. From being an ailment that was associated with many vague causes and reasons, it has now become a medically renowned area of constant research.

It has been asserted throughout this literature that Collapsed Lung is one of those Pulmonology conditions that can be very spontaneous in nature. Hence, its onset cannot be predicted precisely. Nonetheless, enough evidence and risk factors have been compiled to guide an average reader and reduce as much uncertainty as possible.

Apart from treatment options and surgical advancement, it is equally important to know the types of Pneumothorax that can affect various age groups. Such information mentally prepares an individual about the steps to take if the signs and symptoms of a collapsed lung are felt.

The importance of contacting a specialist Pulmonologist can never be stressed enough. While general surgery is capable of treating this condition, the insight that an expert provides is valuable and irreplaceable. Therefore, even if the attack is minor in magnitude, do not take it lightly. Always go to the best and most equipped facilities to ensure that you are given the highest quality treatment.

If you are living with Collapsed Lung, how is your quality of life? Are you satisfied with the way your body feels or are you always scared that the painful condition may recur? No doubt, going through an episode of Pneumothorax not only leaves physical scars, it also affects an individual mentally and emotionally because going through surgery and seeing your body cripple is not easy.

A guide like this, compiled to give you the most basic and essential information in easy terms, helps you deal with Collapsed Lung in a much better way. The kind of activities you should perform, those that you should avoid and the aftercare tips to keep in mind are an asset for patients and caregivers alike, because it improves their understanding of the ailment and gives a guideline to follow from the minute patients are brought out of surgery.

Lastly, this text also provides an insight into the world of those who have experienced Pneumothorax personally. These experiences have been highlighted in great detail to give the average reader an idea of what Pneumothorax can be like.

Be it a celebrity or a stay-at-home mother of three, patient testimonials help because they tell you how others have coped and how you can also do so by following the best practices of pre- and post-surgery care.

Index

Index

www.ingramcontent.com/pod-product-compliance
Lightning Source LLC
Chambersburg PA
CBHW051726170526
45167CB00002B/817